H
TAKE CONTOL OF YOUR OWN LIFE

A Self-Help Guide to Becoming Healthier Over the Next 30 Days

Series 3

CATHY HARRIS

Angels Press, Atlanta, GA
http://www.AngelsPress.com

Published By:
Angels Press
P.O. Box 5288
Atlanta, GA 31107
Phone: (770) 873-2072
http://www.angelspress.com
info@angelspress.com

Copyright © 2013 Cathy Harris
All rights reserved.
ISBN: 1484093364
ISBN-13: 9781484093368

No part of this book may be reproduced in whole or in part, in any form or by any means, electronic or mechanical, including photocopying, recording or by any information storage and retrieval system, without permission in writing from the author.

ATTENTION UNIVERSITIES, COLLEGES, AND PROFESSIONAL ORGANIZATIONS: Quantity discounts are available in bulk purchases of this book for educational and gift purposes. Special books or book excerpts can also be created to fit specific needs. For information, please contact Angels Press, P.O. Box 5288, Atlanta, GA 31107, Phone: (770) 873-2072, http://www.angelspress.com, info@angelspress.com.

Book Cover: Torrie Cooney
http://www.TorrieCooney.blogspot.com

DEDICATION

This book is dedicated to everyone who is seeking to become a healthier and more energized person. You can heal yourself starting within the next 30 days. I am living proof of that!

This book is also dedicated to my two lovely daughters who bounced back even though I raised them eating the very foods and living in the type of environment, I am speaking against today. Keep moving forward ladies, you have made me very, very proud!

ACKNOWLEDGMENTS

I want to dedicate this book to my friends and acquaintances that have passed on due to health issues. Because of them, I set out on this journey to educate myself, my family and the entire community on how to become healthier starting in 30 days or less.

It's because of their sacrifices that many will understand how they can live a full and more productive life. They will never be forgotten!

CONTENTS

Dedication	iii
Acknowledgments	iv
Introduction	vii
Preface	ix
Disclaimer	xvii

1 Detoxify Your Body (Colon, Liver, Kidneys) — 1
-What is Detoxification?
-First Stage of Detoxification – "Your Colon"
-Second Stage of Detoxification – "Your Liver"
-Third Stage of Detoxification – "Your Kidneys"

2 What You Need to Know About Genetically Modified Organisms and the Food Supply System — 20
-The Devastating Effects of Eating Genetically Modified Organisms (GMOs)
-Why You Should Grow Your Own Garden
-What Cooked Foods Are Doing to Your Body

3 Take the Right Vitamin and Mineral Supplements — 37
-What are Vitamins and Minerals?
-How to Find the Right Supplements
-The Immune System is Vital to Your Existence

4 Fasting is Good for You — 44
-What is Fasting?
-How Long Should You Fast?
-Why You Should Engage in Juicing

5 Stay Away from Meat — 50
-What You Really Need to Know About Eating Meat
-Why You Should See the Food Inc. Movie
-How To Keep Down Inflammation in Your Body

6 Chew Your Food — 56
-The Correct Way to Eat Foods
-Is it Heartburn or Indigestion?

7	**Stop Eating Mucus-Producing Foods** -Reasons You Should Avoid Dairy Products -Why You Should Avoid Processed Foods -Pay Attention to Your Allergies	58
8	**Constantly Expel Toxins Out of Your Body** -Ways to Expel Toxins from Your Body -Hot and Cold Sitz Baths	70
9	**Drink the Right Type of Water** -What is the Right Type of Water? -Causes of Dehydration -Stop Drinking Tap Water	73
10	**Stop Taking Pharmaceuticals** -Long Term Effects of Medications -Know Your Numbers and Save Your Life -Recommended List of Yearly Examinations	78
11	**Get Some Type of Cardiovascular Exercise** -Couch Potato Lifestyle -What to Do Before Starting an Exercise Program -The Right Way to Lose Weight	93
12	**Get Plenty of Rest** -Keep a Regular Sleep Schedule -Make Your Bedroom Sleep Friendly	101

About the Author

INTRODUCTION

Have you been feeling sick, sluggish or run-down? Do you consider yourself to be healthy? What does being healthy really means? Being healthy is simply having the energy and vitality to move forward and enjoy your life.

After conducting extensive research on how to become healthier, I learned that it's a good chance that all the following have contributed to your organs becoming clogged, turning hard and slowing you down -- eating the Standard American Diet (SAD) over the years; Swallowing undigested foods over the years; Eating junk foods over the years; and taking pharmaceuticals (either prescribed or over-the-counter) over the years – just to name a few.

Even though you are not experiencing any pain from your liver, kidneys or other organs, it doesn't mean that they are operating at 100%. The problem is if you don't do something to reverse the damage that has occurred to your organs over the years, they will eventually give out. If one organ gives out, they all will give out because they work as a team -- and you will die!

If you have bad breath, pass gas that has a foul odor or have a bad odor when you defecate, that means you have something inside of you that is dying or in other words, a disease is developing in your body.

Remember diseases cannot exist in a healthy body. The goal is to look at your lifestyle (diet, exercise, sleep patterns, etc.) and your environment (inside environment and outdoor environment) and develop good habits that will give you a disease-free body.

Don't beat yourself up if it takes some time for you to adjust to your new lifestyle. After all you did not pick up all those bad habits overnight.

Remember, it takes 3 to 4 weeks to form new habits. But you have to start today before it's too late! Also remember chances are you are the cause and you will also have to be the cure for what is happening to your body.

This is a self-help guide to renewing your life and getting back the energy and vitality you had years ago and I am living proof that you can do this and more starting within the next 30 days.

This book *"How To Take Control of Your Own Life: A Self-Help Guide to Becoming Healthier Over the Next 30 Days"* is the **third book** in a 3-part empowerment book series which provides powerful information on how to take control of your own life. Good luck!

PREFACE – A NOTE TO THE READER

A few months after I lost two of my best friends to cancer, I set out on a journey to educate myself about the disease and how to stop it from taking other people that I deeply cared about.

I eventually discovered that most people had no idea what was going on when it came to their health. Many of us push our own health problems to the background and we engage in overwhelming activities in order to help and assist others.

But you can't help others unless you help your ownself, so your motto should be *"Self, Family* and *Community."*

During the time when my friends died, I had no idea that my life too would become a struggle to survive. When I turned 50 years old, my body gave out on me. It totally shut down and I eventually became housebound and then bed-ridden.

My mom had lived until the age of 82 and so had her mom. But why had I met such a different fate?

I thought about all the things I still wanted to do with my life, the places I wanted to go, the people I wanted to see, and the legacies I still wanted to leave to my grandkids and their kids, etc. It was all now too late for me, "I thought!"

The thought of it all being over was very agonizing! I literally thought I was dying! I knew that people had come back from illnesses and went on to do great things with their lives but because the pain was so bad, I knew it would not be my story.

This book is not just about cancer but it's about every disease and illness in America and how diseases and illnesses are formed in the first place.

After my friend's death, I soon learned that cancer deaths and many other diseases are not only preventable but they are also curable.

After my second friend died, I too fell ill. For weeks I had noticed a feeling of sluggishness as my energy slowly drained from my body. I soon noticed I had stopped going out of the house and was eventually becoming housebound.

At first I thought my energy decrease and feeling of sluggishness was about my friends, I thought I was grieving! But after the New Year rolled around, I knew it was much more than just grieving for my friends.

I was convinced that I was heading on some type of collision course with some type of illness or disease which would eventually take my life like my friends.

The pain started off as a small uncomfortable pain that went from my lower back to my stomach area to my knees. Simple things such as going for my daily power walks and mopping the floor became hard to do because of the back pain.

Over time, it had become an excruciating pain which lasted for up to 5 to 6 hours a day -- everyday. Being a person with a low tolerance for pain, I quickly sought out help from 6 doctors including 2 specialists.

For weeks, I pulled myself out of my home and went to these doctors and specialists waiting to hear the bad news that it was too late for me.

The daily pain was so bad, it did not matter if I stood up or laid down, there was no stopping this excruciating pain! I could have easily called an ambulance to be taken to the hospital but what good would that do?

I was already seeing all these health professionals who were telling me over and over that I was fine, that there was nothing wrong with me.

Everyday when I got out of bed, my only goal was to get back in bed because my pH balance was off, which I later learned, meant my body was extremely toxic. During this time, I almost became bed-ridden.

Not only was I too dizzy to go for my daily walks but getting in and out of the bathtub also proved to be a challenge. As the pain kept growing, the health professionals relayed to me that all my tests, still proved negative for any type of illness or disease.

When the last health professional, an OB GYN Specialist, told me I was fine with no signs of cancer or anything to be concerned about, I could have literally jumped out of the chair because the pain was so terrible. I could not believe it! I just wanted an answer to what was happening to me and my body!

After the last doctor's visit, I went home and really reevaluated what was happening to me. I decided right then and there, that if I was going to stop this pain inside of me and save my life, then it would strictly be up to me.

The medical profession had failed me. Doctors with degrees and a lifetime of cures for others could not figure out what was wrong with me. They could not stop the excruciating pain! All I wanted was for the suffering to stop!

Next, I sat down at the computer and went on Amazon.com where I usually ordered my books to conduct research on certain topics that I wanted to know more about.

Had I not been such a good researcher, I know for a fact that I probably would not be here today! I then ordered over 100 books at one sitting. I wanted answers! And I wanted them fast, before it was too late! I wanted to save my life but I was not sure I could do it!

I ordered books on *"How the Body Works; Exercising; Nutrition; Raw Foods; Organic Foods; Processed Foods; Cancer; Diseases; Parasites; Heavy Metals; Toxic Body"* – just to name a few.

During this time not only did I buy books online but I bought books from local bookstores and checked out tons of health books from the health and fitness section in several local community libraries.

I was on a race against time and if I did not act as soon as possible, it would be too late for me. With the last bit of energy draining from my body, I knew I was at the "eleventh hour" of my situation.

So I shut down and read the books. If the books could not tell me what to do, then I needed to prepare myself and my family because my life would be over at the age of 50.

As I read the books, I took breaks and went through all my personal belongings, got my will in order and organized everything, in case these were the last days of my life. At the time I ran a business which I had to close down until I recuperated.

While reading the books the information was all the same. The first step the books told me to do was to take myself off all processed foods (anything in boxes, cans, packages, jars, etc.) and eat only fresh, raw, organic foods – blended, juiced or steamed -- only.

For a person who had eaten cooked foods her whole life, it was a hard transition but I knew I had to do it to save my life!

I found a neighborhood farmer's market and went "cold turkey" off all processed foods. I blended, juiced or steamed at least 80% of what I ate daily.

I learned quickly that *"Your Health Begins in Your Colon."* The goal was for me to start having at least 2 or 3 easy bowel movements a day. I quickly found out that if you have a toxic bowel, it could cause pain to show up in any area of your body.

As I looked in the mirror daily, I saw how dull my face looked, with no glow or shine in it like it had in the past. My body had changed right before my eyes!

My fingernails had turned totally black, and a nurse who I met in a store, not a medical doctor, had commented by looking at them that I had heavy metals in my body.

As I read more about heavy metals in the body, it just all made sense that that was one of the things that was happening to my body.

When I started implementing the changes the books talked about, the pain started subsiding or disappearing. I began to get more energy to do even more research and I even started back walking again.

I felt I was onto something. It was like some type of "awakening." I could not believe the pain started going away and I realized I was actually healing my own body.

I also read that pH balance meant that my body was real toxic and the only way to get rid of the toxicity was to clean out my organs starting with my colon, liver and kidneys, which are the detoxification organs of the entire body.

I realized that the body products (soaps, lotions, perfumes, etc.) and cleaning products that I was using in my home was toxic and full of toxins, and the way that toxins enters your body was through the air you breathe, the water you drink and food you eat.

I then realized that walking everyday and breathing in the car fumes which are also toxins had also contributed to my body shutting down, so I found a park to walk in.

I joined a gym again and realized when I sat in the sauna in the past, I had always felt better afterwards. At that time I did not realize I was actually releasing toxins from my body.

I learned that I had been drinking the wrong type of water all these years and thought back about the summer the doctor diagnosed me on 5 different occasions with being dehydrated.

Even though he told me I was dehydrated and that I was drinking the wrong type of water, the doctor NEVER told me what type of water to drink because he did not know the answer. I begin to realize that doctors did not know everything and had very little training on nutrition.

After 30 days the pain was down to a few minutes instead of a few hours and the glow to my skin and fingernails returned slowly along with my energy.

Then I found a health food store with a good colon, liver and kidney detox and took each detox back-to-back for an entire year, and then the rest is history.

Remember a symptom can never disappear if you don't remove the original cause. So I had to get to the root of the pain. It just all made sense why my body shut down on me at the age of 50.

No one can get away with eating and drinking anything they want just because it tastes good and they are young. Just like no one can get away with living and working in a toxic environment and putting toxic products on their bodies.

I remembered how I had partied in my 20s, lived and worked in toxic environments in my 30s and 40s which all had contributed to my body shutting down when I turned 50.

At some point we have to take responsibility for our health and well-being. But you have to do it before your body shut down on you! You have to do it before it is too late!

The newfound information was a godsend to me. I was already exercising, but my new way of eating has completely transformed my life, physically, mentally and spiritually.

For those of you who have totally put yourself in the hands of your doctors, or if you want to rejuvenate or renew your life before it's too late, then you need to read my story, my health testimony, and take the 12 steps outlined in the 12 chapters of this book.

This book is my living testimony about how you can heal your own self and save your own life and I am living proof of that. Good luck!

WARNING - DISCLAIMER

This book is provided to help anyone who has been feeling sick, sluggish or run-down. It is a step-by-step guide to provide steps on how to gain the vitality and energy that you need to rejuvenate and renew your life. The author is not in the medical profession but she is a health and wellness expert.

The information provided is intended for educational purposes only. It is not meant to either directly or indirectly give medical advice or prescribe treatment. Please consult with your physician or other licensed health care professional for medical diagnosis, prescription, and treatment.

CHAPTER 1
DETOXIFY YOUR BODY
(Colon, Liver, and Kidneys)

What Is Detoxification?

We have all heard about the role of detoxification in creating great health. Many of us have experienced the detox process, some by attending a health retreat designed for this purpose, and some by virtue of a supervised fast or cleansing program initiated by a naturopathic or holistic practitioner.

But what exactly is detoxification, and what is happening in the body when we engage in this type of specialized program? Detoxification (detox for short) is the physiological or medicinal removal of toxic substances from the human body.

Detoxification is a natural healing process needed more than ever in today's toxic world. With the onslaught of chemicals in our food, air and water, we can all do with undergoing a specific program of periodic cleansing.

Just as the outer environments in which we live can become polluted with trash, violated with industrial chemicals, and covered in sickness-causing smog, our inner environments (our bodies) can become filled with toxic garbage as well.

Many of these toxins come from our diets, drug use, and environmental exposure, both acute and chronic. Internally, free radicals and other irritating molecules act as toxins.

Poor digestion, colon sluggishness and dysfunction, reduced liver function, and poor elimination through the kidneys, respiratory tract, and skin, all add to increased toxicity.

Detoxification involves dietary and lifestyle changes which reduce the intake of toxins and improve elimination. Avoidance of chemicals, from food or other sources, refined food, sugar, caffeine, alcohol, tobacco, and many drugs helps minimize the toxin load. Those lifestyle changes are a direct result of choices you make in your life.

By engaging in a detoxification program, we are actively assisting and supporting the body in its own natural cleansing actions, to help in ridding the body of substances that may be detrimental to our health.

Organic fruits and vegetables are essentially good for detoxification. The goal is to begin to transition to a diet rich in fresh, raw, organic fruits and vegetables with very few cooked or processed foods, to help keep your digestive system free of mucus plaque.

The goal is *"bad stuff out and good stuff in."* Regular and easy elimination will be the rule. Toxins will not build up and foods will be fully digested and utilized.

Detox diets are hard to start but at the end you will have more energy and vitality. Since it was a process of years or decades to get the body so full of plaque and toxins, it will be a process to detoxify and get your body pure and back to its highest possible state of health.

Detoxes are also referred to as *"body cleansers"* and you need to engage in different ones several times a year.

Three detoxes you should engage in include:
1. **Colon Detox:** A good colon detox (also referred to as "*intestinal detox*") might be from 2, to 3, to 4 weeks. This is the MOST IMPORTANT detox which you should do at least twice or 3 times a year. It depends on your diet.
2. **Liver Detox:** This detox can be for 30 days or longer. You should do this detox at least twice a year.
3. **Kidney Detox:** This detox can be for 30 days or longer. Try to stay away from meat during this detox. You should do this detox at least twice a year.

How Sicknesses and Diseases Are Formed in the First Place

According to many holistic healers, it's all about balance. It turns out that the single measurement most important to your health is the pH of your blood and tissues, how alkaline or acidic it is. Different areas of the body have different ideal pH levels, but blood pH is the most telling of all.

The blood must be kept in very narrow pH range, mildly basic or alkaline. If your body is too acidic, it corrodes body tissue, and if left unchecked will interrupt all cellular activities and functions which will interfere with life itself.

The goal is to eat a proper balance of alkaline and acid foods. That means 80 percent of your diet must be alkalizing foods, like green organic vegetables (mostly raw). That percentage can go down once you balance your body.

Just as our body temperature must be maintained at 98.6 degrees Fahrenheit, our blood is ideally maintained at 7.365 pH. You can get the pH of your blood checked with a doctor, wholistic practitioner or you can buy the pH strips at any drug store.

You can test your saliva or urine. The urine can provide the best estimate of what's happening but it is not always right. Blood pH is more reliable, and thus a better indicator of internal conditions of your body.

Everyone should sit down with a naturopathic or holistic specialist, practitioner or healer especially a kinesiologist who specializes in analyzing blood at least once in their lives.

These specialists can look at your blood and tell you exactly what is happening in your body. If you are at risk for a disease, then they can tell by looking at "dry" and "live" blood samples.

In the early stages of imbalance, the symptoms may not be very intense and include such things as skin eruptions, headaches, allergies, colds and flu, and sinus problems.

As things get further out of whack, more serious situations arises. Weakened organs and systems start to give way, resulting in dysfunctional thyroid glands, adrenals, liver, and so on.

If tissue pH deviates too far to the acid side, oxygen levels decrease and cellular metabolism will stop. In other words, cells die. You die!

Chronic symptoms show up when all possibilities of neutralizing or eliminating acid have been exhausted. The imbalance in the blood pH leads to irritation and inflammation and set the stage for sickness.

For example, the body may throw off acids through the skin, producing symptoms such as eczema, acne, boils, headaches, muscle cramps, soreness, swelling, irritation, inflammation, and general aches and pains.

Heart disease is the number one killer in the U.S. with Cancer being number two and Diabetes number three. Diabetes is the number one killer of African Americans so you should read my article *"Diabetes 101: The Number One Killer of African Americans"* and my book on cancer *"Cancer Cures: Heal Your Body and Save Your Life"* at http://www.AngelsPress.com.

First Stage of Detoxification – "Your Colon"

If you don't get anything else out of this book, remember that *"Your Heath Begins in Your Colon!"* In fact, the road to health begins with colon/intestinal cleansing and detoxification, no matter what the disease or problem.

There's been quite a bit of debate about colon cleansing in recent years. People who do it swear by it. They're often walking testimonials of the disease that can be swept from the body in this manner.

But people who've never done it can think colon cleansing sounds a bit strange, and really, who can blame them? However, it's a fact that common 21st century diets are largely abnormal for the human species and this is why colon cleansing is so important in this day and age.

Colon cleansing has become a favorite technique of many successful holistic healers and naturopaths around the world. Bowel movements are the basis of your health. If you don't have at least one bowel movement per day, you are already walking your way toward disease.

Natural Colon Cleansing
A healthy colon weighs 1 to 4 pounds. A proper colon cleanse and detoxification program prepares your body for optimal health by removing the mucus plaque from your colon.

Colon cleanse, Bowel Cleanse, Intestinal Cleanse or *Intestinal Therapy* are terms referring to a procedure (or a therapy) which has as its main goal having a clean bowel.

A good bowel cleanse can take from 2, 3, to 4 weeks up to a few months, depending on the person. But don't get discouraged, it's worth it!

Natural colon cleansing means following a colon cleansing diet along with taking some colon cleansing supplements which may include herbs which are known to kill parasites and worms; contain digestive enzymes; contain probiotics (beneficial bacteria); contain herbs that stimulates the liver, gallbladder and intestines; contain psyllium husk or seeds; contain products like bentonite clay which bind toxins; or cleansers such as enemas or colonic irrigation.

A lot of toxins are excreted through the bowel, so a well-functioning moving bowel is an essential part of any detox program. By cleansing and supporting the bowel in this way, we ensure the maximum removal of toxic substances.

You can buy a good herbal colon cleanse at health food stores. I enjoy the full-body colon cleanse, *CleanStart*, at "Nature's Sunshine" (NaturesSunshine.com) or the colon cleanse at "Renew Life" (RenewLife.com).

When and after detoxifying your colon, it is also important to incorporate probiotics in your diet to replenish your intestinal flora.

You can buy probiotics from a health food store or off health websites and you probably want to keep probiotics in a refrigerator. It's especially important to take daily probiotics when you are on any type of medication.

Causes of Constipation

One of the most frequent bowel problems that people experience today is constipation. A constipated system is one in which the transition time of toxic wastes is slow. The longer the transit time, the longer the toxic waste matter sits in your bowel, and turns into disease.

Constipation may also be a side-effect of iron supplements, pain killers and antidepressants. Even with one bowel movement per day, you will still have at least three meals worth of waste matter rotting or decaying in your colon at all times.

Two easy bowel movements per day are recommended and if you have three movements, then you are really on the right path. Man's body has not changed very much in the past several thousand years, however, man's diet has certainly changed a lot.

All the refined sugar, white flour, hormone/antibiotic-filled meats, we constantly ingest constitute an assault on our bodies. In other words, we are continuously violating our bodies by eating the Standard American Diet (SAD).

The thing about a chemical-oriented, processed, highly-sugared and heavy meat-eating diet is that our bodies aren't equipped to process all of those things, and if we can't process them, often times we can't eliminate them.

This means that old fecal matter gets stuck inside our bodies and becomes corroded on our colon walls. In a nutshell, this is why constipation is common and drug companies sell 1.5 billion dollars' worth of laxatives each year.

After years or decades of accumulation, it can lead to disease in the colon, or anywhere in the body. The colon walls are full of pores and what is trapped inside the colon will eventually leak into the blood where it can be transported to accumulate anywhere in the body.

Where it accumulates will often be the deciding factor as to the symptoms, or disease, your body develops.

Digestive disorders caused by slow moving bowel movements include constipation, hemorrhoids, irritable bowel syndrome, colitis, and crohn's disease – just to name a few.

Other diseases that have been related to the bowels include diabetes, gall stones, kidney stones, gout, hypertension, varicose veins, rheumatoid arthritis, psoriasis, and obesity.

For constipation eat foods with fiber especially fresh, raw, organic, green vegetables, exercise regularly and drink plenty of water. You should also stop eating all forms of pasta (spaghetti, ravioli, roman noodles, etc.) which acts like a glue in your intestines.

Chronic Yeast Infections and Toxic Bowels
Today, matters are made even worse because most of the population also lives with a common fungal condition

called "*candida*" or "*candidiasis*" overgrowth (yeast). More and more doctors are now aware of how chronic yeast infections such as candida are caused by toxic bowels.

Bacteria, yeast, fungus, and mold do not themselves produce symptoms in the body, their toxic wastes do. Nor do they initiate disease. They only show up because of a compromised environment.

General signs of an overgrowth of yeast include chronic fatigue (especially after eating), depression, bloating, gas, cramps, chronic diarrhea or constipation, rectal itching, allergies, severe PMS, impotence, memory loss, severe mood swings, recurrent fungal infections (such as athlete's foot), extreme sensitivity to chemicals (perfumes, smoke, odors, etc.), and lightheadedness or drunkenness after minimal wine, beer, or sugar – just to name a few.

One of the most well-known forms of yeast is the "*vaginal yeast infection*." A vaginal yeast infection is irritation of the vagina and the area around it called the vulva. This infection may play a role in just about any mental health condition or chronic illness you can think of.

Candida is inside all of us. It normally resides in the intestinal tract, mouth, throat and genitals, however, it can burrow holes in the intestinal tract, enter the blood stream and then make its way into any organ of the body. To make matters worse it discharges over 70 different toxins into the body.

Although we're actually supposed to have small amounts of candida in our colon, candida overgrowth becomes a problem when the healthy bacteria in our colons are killed.

This is commonly done with chemicals in our diets, chlorine in our water, antibiotics doled out like candy, steroid medications and birth control pills. When we no longer have our healthy bacteria to keep the candida in small proportions, the candida yeast grows to large proportions.

Candida leads to pollution in the body, not just in the colon, but throughout the entire body and it's a primary cause of disease. Getting rid of candida is always tough. In fact, if you have a serious overgrowth, it can be very, very tough.

As a matter of fact, beating cancer is faster and easier. If you have been suffering from candida yeast infections for years, finding little success using diet or drugs or herbal products, you know how hard it is to eliminate.

Second Stage of Detoxification – "Your Liver"

These days most people don't know much about their liver, except perhaps that alcohol damages it. Most people don't know how to care for this all important organ either. Your liver is a hardworking three to five pound organ that sits under your right rib cage.

It's about the size of a football. Unlike most organs with just a handful of jobs in your body, your liver has over a thousand jobs, and daily detoxification is one of its most important ones.

Your liver is your prime detoxification organ. It's responsible for rendering harmless the hundreds of man-made chemicals that most people put in and on their bodies each and every week. It takes pollutants out of the bloodstream, identifies them and alters them into safer substances to be excreted via the organs of elimination.

This process is always happening automatically, just like when we breathe and our hearts beat. It's not something we need to think about on a day to day basis. It is a natural state of the body to be continually cleansing, and most of the time we don't even notice it is happening.

It is estimated that there are 50,000+ chemicals in production, with 10,000 of these used in food processing. With the amount of potentially harmful chemicals in our environment, our food, our personal care and cleaning products, in air and water pollution, and in recreational drugs and medications that many people take, our body's burden of toxic substances can rise.

When the liver is unable to deal with an excessive amount of circulating toxins, they can continue to move through the body. This causes disruption and damage, before eventually being stored mainly in the fat cells of our organs and tissues, often being stored for years or decades.

When your liver is overwhelmed with incoming chemicals, two things happen:
1. First, those chemicals and toxins back up in your body and become trapped inside because your liver didn't have the resources to deal with them. When there is an accumulation of these chemicals and toxins in your body, health problems are often the result.
2. Second, weight loss becomes difficult because in addition to being your prime detoxification organ, your liver is your prime "_fat burning organ._" When your liver is overwhelmed with toxins, weight loss can be extremely challenging.

Your Liver and Anger Problems
In Chinese medicine, most organs are connected to an emotion, and your liver is the organ connected to *"anger."* As a society, we see the effects of this quite clearly, but often are unaware of what we're seeing.

If you end up with a toxic liver, it leads to anger problems and to people who have problems controlling or letting go of their anger. Obviously, the more toxic the habits, the worse the situation become.

Habits that take this to the extreme include smoking, taking drugs, and regularly eating junk or processed foods. Studies have also been conducted to see if this is also a reason why many people commit violent crimes and end up in the prison system in this country, from having a toxic liver and not being able to control their anger.

How Chemicals Are Absorbed Into Your Body
Do you know that what you put on your skin, scalp, eyes and gums are absorbed straight into your body's organs, tissues, cells and even the brain? This include foods, cosmetics, toiletries, soaps, perfume, as well as general household products.

Put simply, we are ingesting and therefore literally eating many substances that are toxic to our systems and that causes our bodies to slow down and in some cases shut down.

The sad truth is that even walking through the aisles of some health food stores, there are still so-called healthy products that contain the same kind of harsh chemicals that are found in most commercial products.

So what can we do to avoid the trap of buying products that we believe to be okay? Simple, before buying and using these products check the ingredients listed.

Be Kind to Your Liver by Using Natural Products

Don't overwork your liver! Remember the liver detoxifies everything that comes into your body from the inside and outside of your home.

In order to heal your body and get more energy and vitality, don't make your liver work harder. Be kind to your liver by going natural.

Living a toxic lifestyle will cause you to die prematurely. But you can reclaim and master your health by going natural or embracing the growing green movement.

But be careful with these new green products because many are toxic especially the new green energy saving light bulbs, shopping bags, cleaning products, etc. However, as we recycle, reuse, and reduce consumption, we can still remove toxic substances from our external and internal environment.

Too many people accept the notion that we can consume processed, pesticide-laced, genetically-altered, preservative and chemical laden foods, and that these foods cause no harm in their body. Even if people don't believe this on a conscious level, eating habits often suggest otherwise.

The goal is to go natural and use organic products for 6 months to a year or longer or at least until you have lost the weight you are trying to lose, obtained the energy and vitality you are trying to regain, or gotten your emotions into check especially since the liver is in charge of *obesity, energy* and *emotions*.

The cleaning aisle at just about any grocery store is stocked with a dizzying array of options and when it comes down to it, there are a lot of expensive, toxic, products crowding the market.

Three of the best natural cleansers that you can clean your entire home with include:
1. **Cold-Pressed Olive Oil:** There are several different types of olive oils. Try to buy the "cold-pressed" (or first cold) olive oils. Uses for olive oil include cooking and putting in salads and other dishes; as natural skin lotion; to dust wood furniture; use when detoxifying your liver, etc.
2. **Baking Soda:** (Buy aluminum free from health food stores). Deodorizes refrigerator; Brush teeth with; Use as natural deodorant; Clean house especially floors, carpets, countertops, bathtubs, toilets, etc.
3. **White Distilled Vinegar:** Clean house especially floors, carpets, countertops, bathtubs, toilets, etc.

The goal is to get rid of everything in your house that smells such as perfume, perfumed soaps and candles, aftershave, deodorants, toothpaste, hair products, body lotions, detergents, air fresheners, cleaning products, etc.

Basically, you need to get rid of _every product_ that has the ingredients containing the letters "PROP" especially these ingredients -- propamide, propacetamide, propyl gallate, calcium proprionate, propanol, isopropyl alcohol. These ingredients allows cancers and other diseases and toxins to enter your body.

The good news is that once you stop taking or using these products and start using natural products (from health food stores), their effects will disappear out of your system (your body) within 5 days and you will start feeling better (more energy), and your body will begin to heal.

Essential oils fall into the category of personal care products, which can be "certified organic." Once certified, body care products can be labeled in one of four ways:
1. "*100% organic*" includes only organically produced ingredients.
2. "*Organic*" must be at least 95% organic. Products in both categories may use the USDA organic seal.
3. Products containing at least 70% organic ingredients can be called "*made with organic ingredients*" but may not use the USDA seal.
4. Finally, any product with "*less than 70% organic ingredients*" cannot use the term organic on the main display label.

To learn more about USDA organic certifications, visit USDA.gov and search national organic program.

Fortunately, as with so many of our problems, nature has provided a solution to our toxic environments.

The solution is simply to cleanse your body and liver to remove the stored toxins from your liver and to reduce your body's toxic load.

In today's chemical driven world, internal body cleansing should be as commonly regarded as washing your hands. A good liver detox program is located in your health food stores or at "Renew Life" (RenewLife.com).

Remember also to take the supplements recommended on the side of the box (FiberSmart, etc.) to help with elimination during the detox process.

Ways to Boost Your Energy
Three reasons we are exhausted include anemia, hypothyroidism, and dietary issues. Since the liver is in charge of energy, a lemon is one of the most powerful foods for supporting the digestive organs especially the liver.

Since a lemon can help to turn on the body's energy and it cleanses and activates the liver, start each day with a glass of warm water (distilled, pure/purified or alkaline) and organic lemon juice. If you have an extremely toxic body, drink water and lemon juice throughout the day.

Giving the liver all the nutrients it needs to perform its daily tasks is one of the most important things you can do to boost your energy. You can also take a daily dose of the herb milk thistle which helps regenerate the liver.

Milk thistle and liver supporting vegetables (broccoli, brussel sprouts, cabbage, cauliflower, artichoke, beetroot (beets), onion, garlic, apples, etc.) are especially needed if you live in a toxic environment (inside or outside of your home); eat a toxic diet of junk or processed foods; drink too much alcohol; have hepatitis or have other issues with your liver.

Third Stage of Detoxification – "Your Kidneys"

Our kidneys need detoxification the most. A proper functioning kidney is associated with longevity as well.

It is believed by the Chinese that our kidneys are the center of all our genetic energy and is passed on to us at the time of birth. This clearly states that the detoxification of our kidneys is imperative and should not be ignored.

The detoxification process of the kidneys involve the ultimate system of filtration in our body to flush out water and other substances; regulate the production of blood cells; maintain the pH levels of the blood; and eliminate toxins from the system.

Kidneys have a major role to play in our well-being. Our kidneys function in a similar way like that of a water filter. It helps in filtering the blood in the body and then removes all the wastes that we do not require.

While detoxifying your kidneys, you need to maintain a proper detox diet. Your first step towards kidney detoxification is to minimize your salt and sugar intake and avoid meat which taxes the kidneys.

Fresh fruit juices can be a great aid in detoxifying your kidneys. The juice of fresh vegetables and fruits act as energizers, cleansers, regenerators and builders of our system, so next to water, these juices are the best way to detoxify our system.

Water is definitely the most essential detoxifying agent for the kidneys and we need to drink ample amounts of it. Cranberry fruit juice is well-recognized as a great detoxifying agent for the kidneys also.

But make sure you use the cranberry fruit juice from health food stores, not grocery stores that contains too much sugar.

Kidney detoxes also helps in healing certain cancer, skin problems, arthritis, high blood pressure, liver problems, fatigue and several other health problems and symptoms.

WARNINGS:
- If you have diabetes, high blood pressure, or a family history of kidney disease, you may be at higher risk for kidney disease.
- When you are close to kidney failure your breath smells like urine. Your urine will be dark.
- With a backache avoid all meats and animal protein until healed because it can put undue pressure on kidneys.
- High doses of the painkiller ibuprofen (advil, nuprin, and others) can lead to kidney dysfunction.
- Lead and other metallic poisons are very harmful to the kidneys.
- Aluminum is excreted through the kidneys and toxic amounts may impair kidney functions.

When it comes to detoxification of the kidneys, I enjoy the RenewLife.com 30-day Kidney detox. You can order it off the website or buy the detox program from health foods stores.

How To Detoxify Heavy Metals

After detoxification of your colon, liver and kidneys, there is a good chance that you might still need to get rid of or detoxify heavy metals from your body. If your knee joints are painful and your back stiff, then you might have heavy metals in your body.

Pesticides, city water, and a lifetime of junk food are only a few of the many causes of your accumulation of heavy metals. Heavy metals, such as mercury, aluminum and lead, exist in the environment and often end up entering the human body.

Mercury seeps into the bloodstream by eating Genetically Modified foods which contains pesticides and herbicides which are heavy metals; your amalgam dental fillings; toothpaste; deodorant; breakfast cereals; ice cream; baking soda; vaccines; toxic cleaning products; toxic body products; new green twisty energy saving light bulbs; pollution in the air – just to name a few.

A heavy metal build-up can result in symptoms such as headaches, fatigue and pain. Excess amounts of heavy metals are linked to diseases such as brain cancer, mental illness, bipolar disorder, depression, memory loss, brain fog, autism, Alzheimers, Parkinson's, Multiple Sclerosis (MS), and other debilitating illnesses especially illnesses dealing with the brain.

After a heavy metal detox, however, heavy metal accumulation decreases and symptoms fade away. When embarking on a heavy metal detoxification program, it is very important to consume a diet that is high in protein.

This is because the sulfur-bearing amino acids present in proteins will help the detoxification process. Never attempt to fast in any way while detoxing from heavy metals.

Other natural additions to the diet that greatly improve the detoxification from heavy metals are organic garlic, cilantro, etc.

You can buy a *"Mercury"* or *"Heavy Metal"* detox from "Renew Life" at Renewlife.com or health food stores. Read the article *"How To Gain Back Your Mental Clarity by Eliminating Heavy Metals"* at http://www.AngelsPress.com.

CHAPTER 2
WHAT YOU NEED TO KNOW ABOUT GENETICALLY MODIFIED ORGANISMS AND THE FOOD SUPPLY SYSTEM

The Devastating Effects of Eating Genetically Modified Organisms (GMOs)

The food supply system in this country is under attack, not by terrorists but your own government. Three U.S. governmental agencies, Food and Drug Administration (FDA.gov), U.S. Department of Agriculture (USDA.gov) and the Environmental Protection Agency (EPA.gov) have all said that foods referred to as *"FrankenFoods" (Genetically Modified Organisms (GMOs))* can be sold on the U.S. market even though these foods are causing a massive decline of health in communities all over the country.

The foods have been on the U.S. market since 1996. The foods are named after *"Frankenstein,"* the monster. We all remember how he was put together. So we are talking about over ninety-percent (90%) of all foods in your neighborhood grocery stores especially all processed foods, contains Genetically Modified Organisms (GMOs).

Most people have been brought up thinking what they purchase from their neighborhood store is safe to eat. This is no longer true since most processed foods contain Genetically Modified ingredients that can have disastrous effects on both animal and human health.

Now-a-days, what you purchase from the corner store might just change your DNA and create symptoms so frightening it may be hard to believe. What is worse is that when you go to the doctor to get help, he/she will tell you what you are experiencing, is all in your head.

Biotech Whistleblowers and even the American Academy of Environmental Medicine (AAEM) released its position paper on Genetically Modified (GM) foods stating that Genetically Modified foods pose a serious health risk.

The AAEM called for a moratorium on Genetically Modified foods, with implementation of immediate long-term safety testing and labeling of Genetically Modified foods. The AAEM is just one of many organizations worldwide calling for these steps to be taken.

FrankenFoods which are Genetically Modified Organisms (GMOs) are also called *"Genetically Engineered"* and *"Genetically Altered"* which is an organism whose genetic material has been altered using genetic engineering techniques.

These techniques, generally known as combining genetic DNA technology, use DNA molecules from different sources, which are combined into one molecule to create a new set of genes.

For instance they mix the DNA of a plant with the DNA of an animal so that it will grow quicker, bigger and stronger, while increasing the longevity of the plant or animal, making it some type of *"superbreed."*

These products have undergone only short term testing to determine their effects on humans and the environment. They use DNA primarily from bacteria and fungus. Remember, bacteria are life-forms and they will find a way to survive.

They mix the pesticides and herbicides into plant seeds and the feed of animals, so they would not have to spray crops but this has resulted in bug resistant crops with super weeds and super bugs.

If you eat these foods there is no way to avoid eating pesticides and herbicides which are poisons and heavy metals which causes brain issues such as brain cancer, mental illness, bipolar disorder, depression, memory loss, brain fog, autism, Alzheimers, Parkinson's, Multiple Sclerosis (MS), etc.

This has resulted in people becoming *"zombie-like"* and for many to live in a *"brain-dead society"* where people can't think for themselves.

Other multiple illnesses caused by GMOs include antibiotic resistance diseases and new diseases such as Morgellon's disease; food allergies; toxins; digestive issues; nutritional issues; organ damage; reproductive disorders and birth effects (such as kids born with smaller brains and low birth weight); miscarriages, infertility or lower sperm counts; immune problems; diabetes; cancer; obesity; blindness; accelerated aging – just to name a few.

Some of the main foods that are involved include corn, soybeans, canola, cottonseed, sugar beets, Hawaiian papaya, zucchini, yellow squash, etc.

Other foods containing GMOs include infant formulas, salad dressings, breads, hamburgers, hotdogs, margarines, mayonnaise, cereals, crackers, cookies, chocolate, candy, fried food, chips, veggie burgers, meat substitutes, ice cream, frozen yogurt, tofu, tamari, soy sauce, soy, cheeses, tomato sauces, protein powders, baking powders, alcohol, vanilla, powered sugars, peanut butter, enriched flour, pasta, etc.

Animals that have been Genetically Modified to save time and money are chickens, pigs, turkeys, etc. What is so alarming is that these Genetically Modified chickens cannot urinate so the urine goes back up in them.

That is why these foods taste so juicy to those consuming them. For an egg to turn into a chicken, it takes a period of just one week. In the past in regular chickens, it took at least three weeks for this process.

New Diseases Caused by Genetically Modified Organisms (GMOs)

It appears that a new disease referred to as "*Morgellon's Disease,*" may be a result of Genetically Modified crops and foods. Morgellons (also called Morgellons disease or Morgellons syndrome) (Morgellons.org), is a name given in 2002 by Mary Leitao to a proposed condition referred to by the Centers for Disease Control and Prevention (CDC.gov) as an unexplained skin disease characterized by a range of skin symptoms -- including crawling, biting, and stinging sensations; finding fibers on or under the skin and sticking out of sores; and persistent skin lesions such as rashes or sores.

The constant feeling of something very much like an insect crawling without stop beneath the skin and unbearable itching are two common symptoms. The symptoms are so unbearable but many have been told by the psychiatry industry that it is "imaginary," so many people have committed suicide as a result.

Current scientific consensus holds that Morgellons is not a new disorder and is instead a new and misleading name for a well-known condition. Most doctors, including dermatologists and psychiatrists, regard Morgellons as a manifestation of known medical conditions, including delusional parasitosis (infestation with or a disease caused by parasites).

Despite the lack of evidence that Morgellons is a distinct condition, the Morgellons Research Foundation and self-diagnosed Morgellon's patients have successfully lobbied members of Congress and the CDC to investigate the proposed condition.

The biggest problem with Genetically Modified foods is our bodies cannot digest these foods and now researchers are finding out that thousands of people are now coming down with Morgellon's Disease.

The first testing ground for GMOs was in India where for the past 10 years over 125,000 farmers have committed suicide after eating GMOs and getting the disease.

They also killed themselves not just because they got Morgellon's Disease but because the GMO crops ruined their soil and land, making it unfit to grow any type of food again, so these farmer's livelihoods' were over.

Over 150 countries have allowed GMOs to enter their markets including Paraguay, China, Brazil, Argentina, Canada, etc. So far Europe and Australia has said "*No to GMOs*" but the U.S. government allowed GMOs to enter this country in 1996.

In many cases the foods will cause long-term health issues that will not only affect your family today but future generations to come especially because the foods changes your DNA makeup.

Monsanto – The Bad Seed

Monsanto is a *"profit-motivated"* company. Michael Taylor use to be an attorney with Monsanto as a client. He then went to work at the Food and Drug Administration (FDA.gov).

Then he went to work at Monsanto as their Vice President. Now he is back at FDA.gov as the "U.S. Food Safety Czar" in charge of FDA's food policies. This is a major conflict of interest!

Monsanto and other powerful corporations are well along in their plans to dominate the world's food supply through genetic engineering. Remember, *"He who owns the seeds, control the world's food supply."*

Besides creating Genetically Modified foods, Monsanto also created <u>Agent Orange</u> (which caused many men to get cancer from the Vietnam War); <u>PCPs</u> (which are poisons that were leaked from the plant in Anniston, AL into the water system and killed everyone who lived around the plant and others who lived miles away came down with cancer); <u>DDTs (Dichlorodiphenyltrichloroethane)</u> (which is an insecticide, toxic to humans and animals when swallowed or absorbed through the skin, that has been banned in the U.S. since 1972); <u>Bovine Growth Hormone (rBGH)</u> (growth hormone found today in all beef, milk, chicken, eggs, etc.); <u>Aspartame</u> (a sugar substitute that is causing an explosion of brain cancers); <u>Roundup Ready Weed Killer</u> (poisonous herbicide which is currently being sprayed on all play grounds, football, baseball, soccer fields, etc., so get ready for an explosion of sick kids).

For decades, the Monsanto Corporation of St. Louis has been slowly dominating the world's supply of seeds for crops. Monsanto has spent over $30 billion in recent years buying numerous U.S. seed companies and now they own up to 90% of all the seed companies in the U.S. including 40% of all U.S. grown crops. As a result, they now control the U.S. seed business.

Monsanto specializes in Genetically Modified (GM) seeds. If consumers, farmers and other interested parties, do not educate themselves now, in another five years, Monsanto will own 100% of all the seeds in the U.S.

These GMO seeds have particular properties that Monsanto has patented. Because Genetically Modified seeds are patented, it is illegal for a farmer to retain seeds from this year's crop to plant next year.

To use these patented seeds, farmers must buy new seeds from Monsanto every year. Thus, a farmer who adopts Genetically Modified seeds and fails to retain a stock of traditional seeds could become dependent upon this corporation.

Farmers do have several lawsuits against Monsanto. However, the *"Monsanto Protection Act"* was passed in April 2013, which stops all lawsuits pending against Monsanto. Since this bill was only a rider, it means they will have to pass the bill again in six months.

The U.S. government is very enthusiastic about these new technologies. From the viewpoint of U.S. foreign policy, Genetically Modified seeds offer a key advantage over traditional seeds. Nations, whose farmers are dependent upon corporations for seeds, might forfeit considerable political independence.

A key component of the U.S. Monsanto plan to dominate world agriculture with Genetically Modified seeds is the *"absence of labeling"* of Genetically Engineered foods.

All U.S. foods must carry labels listing the ingredients, salt, sugar, water, vitamins, additives, etc. However, three separate U.S. government agencies have ruled that Genetically Modified foods deserve an exception, they can be sold without being labeled Genetically Modified (GM).

While all this is going on, the FDA is making every effort to prevent the public from knowing the truth about GMOs. They've claimed that requiring Genetically Modified foods to be accurately labeled would be confusing to consumers.

The upshot is that they have no intention to require mandatory Genetically Modified Organisms (GMOs) labeling of food products and in fact the FDA seems committed to making sure consumers are left in the dark.

This strategy has successfully prevented consumers from exercising informed choices in the marketplace, reducing the likelihood of a consumer revolt. But now we need to spread the word throughout the world.

Children and Genetically Modified Organisms (GMOs)
Children face the greatest risk from the potential dangers of Genetically Modified foods for the same reasons they face the greatest risk from other hazards like pesticides and radiation.

These young, fast-developing bodies are influenced most because children's immune systems are not fully developed; Children are more susceptible to allergies; Children are more susceptible to problems with milk;

Children are more susceptible to nutritional problems; and children are in danger from antibiotic resistant diseases.

Pregnant and nursing women must be careful to avoid GMOs at all times. Feeding their children organic baby food including milk provides peace of mind and ensures that they have given their baby the best start.

It is unclear which foods contribute to behavior problems especially in children but remember *"You Are What You Eat!"* Foods can have a profound effect on your behavior, mood, happiness, and your entire quality of life.

Other issues with children include -- One out of 6 kids are learning disabled; Over 60 to 70% of kids are dropping out of school in some areas because of their inability to think, learn and act; Over 60% of kids that graduate from high school are reading at a 6th grade level; Over 25% of kids have Attention Deficit Hyperactivity Disorder (ADHD); Over 75% of kids by age 3 will have ear infections because of being allergic to dairy products and other foods; Kids ages 8-10 years old have diabetes and high blood pressure and are on medications; Kids ages 13 years old have the same veins, arteries, and capillaries as a 45 year old; and over 80% of kids that are overweight will become overweight adults.

Increased rates of obesity are thought to play a major role in early puberty and girls having breasts and periods at age 6 and 7 because body fat can produce sex hormones.

Non-GMO Campaigns
Our 3 step plan of action for our Non-GMO Campaigns include:
1. **_Help Spread the Word:_** Help us spread the word to everyone you know. Our non-GMO campaigns are

targeting healthcare practitioners, patient advocacy and support groups, parents, schools, campuses, youth, health-conscious consumers, natural products industry, media and messaging, chefs and food service industries, etc.

2. **Switch to Organic Foods:** Tell everyone you know to switch to *"100 Certified Organic Foods,"* from organic food co-ops, farmer's markets, other organic health venues or grow foods your own self. If the labels states the foods are *"100% Certified Organic,"* then it's 100% organic and okay to eat. Ideally this is what you want for your family.

But remember, most of the labels of the foods in farmer's markets and other organic health venues states the foods are organic, which means the foods are only 95% organic and 5% is Genetically Modified Organisms (GMOs).

If the foods are labeled *"Containing Organic Ingredients"* then only 70 to 75% of the foods are organic and 25 to 30% contains GMOs.

3. **Contact Your Legislators:** If people knew their foods are Genetically Modified, they would not buy it. So contact your legislators from the ground up and ask them to introduce and pass bills to label foods as Genetically Modified (GM).

Join us on Facebook.com for the *"National Non-GMO Health Movement"* that I launched and read my blog at http://NonGMOHealthMovement.blogspot.com.

Learn more about the *"Campaign for Healthier Eating in America"* by Jeffrey Smith and read his book *"Seeds of*

Deception" (SeedsofDeception.com). His other websites are http://www.ResponsibleTechnology.org and http://www.NonGMOShoppingGuide.com.

Other Non-GMO campaigns you need to know about include – *Food Integrity Program* at the Government Accountability Project (GAP); *Occupy Monsanto* (Occupy-Monsanto.com); *Millions Against Monsanto* (http://www.MillionsAgainstMonsanto.org); *Genetically Modified (GM) Watch* (GMWatch.org); *Food and Water Watch* (FoodandWaterWatch.org) – just to name a few.

Why You Should Grow Your Own Garden

We can protect our health and the environment by making healthier non-GMO choices. You can buy food from farmer's markets, whole food and health food stores, as well as peddlers from the side of the road, but the only way to insure that the foods are "*100% Certified Organically Grown*" is to grow it yourself in your own gardens.

Every household need their own organic garden or grow a garden at a relative or friends' home or join a food co-op. Families must come together now for the sake of future generations.

Edible gardening is a growing trend. Millions of households grow vegetables, fruits, berries or herbs. The reasons you should grow your own garden include to save money on your food bill and to grow foods you know is safe.

Wholefoods stores have admitted that 70% of their foods are organic which means 30% is not. So if you buy foods from these types of establishments, you need to find new organic venues to buy your foods. It is even rumored that Monsanto own a line of wholefood stores.

To deter others from starting organic farms, the government, FDA.gov, is charging outrageous fees and/or forcing farmers to buy Genetically Modified Monsanto seeds only. They are also making it illegal to grow, share, trade and sell homegrown food. There are business owners or groups in every city that will help you learn how to grow your own garden so seek them out today.

Organic vs. Non-Organic
The most healthful fruits and vegetables are those that have been grown organically, without the use of insecticides, herbicides, artificial fertilizers, or growth-stimulating chemicals and especially GMOs.

Also remember that organic foods spoils quicker, so it might be necessary to shop more often for your food. But the benefits in the long run will be worth it because eating organic means you will cut down on doctor's visits.

The new rules do not allow a crop to be called organic if it is Genetically Modified. But organic certification does not require GMO tests. If the seeds when purchased were described by the seller as a non-GMO and if the farming and production methods were designed to exclude GMOs, then the product may pass "organic certification."

Remember with a strong wind, seeds from GMO crops can travel up to a half of mile and affect a non-GMO crop. So the seeds might have been contaminated, the crops cross-pollinated, or accidental mixing after harvest might have gone undetected.

However, the product may still be labeled as organic, just as long as the producer and certifier doesn't know about the contamination. This put organic producers in an uncomfortable bind.

If you don't have access to organic foods like many people up north then buy the regular kind and wash the food off with just plain water. Many of the food washers contains unhealthy ingredients. If fresh produce is unavailable, use frozen foods but always try to stay away from frozen or canned foods.

One thing the experts agree on, regardless of whether you choose locally grown, organic, or conventional foods, the important thing is to eat plenty of produce. Health experts recommend eating a variety of fruits and vegetables so you can take advantage of their diverse nutritional benefits. But remember be careful eating fruits which contain the bad sugars, which turns acidic in your body.

Learn to "Eat to Live" vs. "Living to Eat"
Moving toward an alkaline lifestyle and diet is a process, not a single event or an overnight transformation. When you *"Eat to Live,"* you eat with awareness.

To maintain a balanced pH in your blood and tissues, your diet should consist of at least 70 to 80% fresh, wholesome, organic foods (at least half should be raw) and no more than 20 to 30 percent acidifying foods.

Most of your foods should be juiced, blended or steamed only. Eight ounces of fresh vegetable juices is an ideal beginning to any meal or an excellent snack. All the benefits of vegetables can be enhanced simply by juicing them.

If you don't have time to juice your foods, make sure you also include green grasses from health food stores in your diet. Wheat grass contains more than one hundred food elements. It is 25 percent protein and has high amounts of an antifungal substance. Barley and Kamut grass is also good for you.

Some alkalizing foods that should be eaten as often as possible and should be ORGANIC include -- asparagus, beets, broccoli, brussels sprouts, burdock, cabbage, carrots, cauliflower, celery, cucumbers, eggplant, garlic, green and yellow squash (zucchini and summer squash), green beans, greens of all kinds (including spinach, mustard greens, collards, kale, lettuce, watercress, and Swiss chard), okra, onions, parsley, parsnips, peas (fresh), radishes, red, yellow and green peppers, rutabagas, salsify, scallions, sea vegetables such as nori, wakame, and hijiki, sprouted grains, seeds, turnips, water chestnuts, etc.

For as long as you are having symptoms or not feeling well, go easy on the high-sugar vegetables such as carrots, beets, and winter squash. Eating broadly at all times will give you the type of nutrients you need to stay healthy.

The goal is to consume foods that will provide you the essential nutrients and enzymes to live a long and healthy life.

People who are *"Living to Eat"* are eating empty calories and starving their bodies of essential nutrients and enzymes.

Without proper nutrition, the body can't heal or regenerate its tissues as necessary. If you can't digest foods, the tissues will eventually starve, which will cause a lack of energy, make you feel sick and accelerate the aging process.

Approximately 20 percent of your calories should come from healthy fats. They are the building blocks of fats that strengthen cell walls.

Polyunsaturated fats such as flax, borage, primrose, grape seed and hemp oils help construct cell membranes, produce hormones, and bind and eliminate acids.

Most oils contain both monounsaturated and polyunsaturated fats, and those that are predominately monounsaturated, such as olive oil (as well as raw nuts and avocados) are also beneficial.

Nuts, seeds, avocados are all good sources of healthy fats including the Omega 3s and 6s. Organic tomatoes and avocados are also good vegetable choices (though technically they are fruits), because eaten raw, they are alkalizing.

You should always eat antioxidants. Antioxidants are natural compounds that help protect the body from harmful free radicals. These are atoms that can damage cells and damage your immune system.

You'll find them in colorful fruits and vegetables especially those with purple, blue, red, orange, and yellow hues. They are especially helpful in fighting cancer.

To get the biggest benefits of antioxidants, eat these foods raw or lightly steamed. Don't overcook or boil antioxidants. If you are not getting enough antioxidants in your diet then take an antioxidant supplement. The three major antioxidant vitamins or supplements are beta-carotene, vitamin C, and vitamin E.

What you also need to remember is that some foods act as medicine in your body while other foods act as a poison. Therefore, you should order and read the book *"Eat Right 4 Your Type"* by naturopathic doctor Dr. Peter J. D'Adamo. This book discusses why certain people with certain blood types should avoid certain foods. Also read his books *"Live Right 4 Your Type"* and *"Cook Right 4 Your Type."*

What Cooked Foods Are Doing to Your Body

Cooked Foods Are Your Body's Enemy
Try to stay away from cooked foods as much as possible. People are walking around tired after a big meal because their bodies respond to cooked foods as a foreign invader, toxin or poison.

Not only does cooking food deplete nutrients, if you eat cooked foods, you are setting yourself up for illnesses and diseases by inviting bacteria, mold, fungus and yeast into your body.

You also want to stay away from molded foods which allow toxins and parasites to enter the body so make sure you are in a position to monitor your food. If your food spoils, throw it out!

Beware of Good Cooks!
Are you a *"Good Cook?"* Every family has one or in many cases two or three. It can be your mother or their mother, an aunt, a cousin or even your daughter. Nowadays being a good cook could mean that you are also unhealthy.

These cooks have continued to use recipes passed down from their ancestors which were made up of all type of unhealthy and fattening ingredients such as flour, sugar, oils, etc., which continues to contribute to tons of obesity and sickness today.

Instead of admitting that these cooks are preparing unhealthy meals for their families, in many communities we continue to praise them.

If we are ever going to stop this explosion of sickness in this country especially in African American families, we need to be truthful about the foods we are preparing in our households.

Throw Out Your Microwave
Good cooks use their stoves and microwaves 100 percent of the time. Because of the economy, people are stressed out, frustrated and overwhelmed with life and many turn to their microwave several times a day to prepare meals for their families.

Using microwaves can be very detrimental to your health. Not only do microwaves causes cancer but if you eat foods that have been microwaved, the foods can continue to cook in your stomachs, damaging your insides.

The goal is to replace your microwaves and stoves with a juicer, blender or steamer and eat foods in as natural forms as possible.

Because cooking destroys those all-important enzymes, the more of your organic vegetables you eat raw, the better. Aim to have at least 40 percent of your food uncooked, working up to 75 to 80 percent.

CHAPTER 3
TAKE THE RIGHT VITAMIN AND MINERAL SUPPLEMENTS

What are Vitamins and Minerals?

If you are eating cooked foods, which depletes nutrients and have no nutritional value, you need to take vitamin and mineral supplements every day.

Vitamins and minerals are essential to life. Vitamins and minerals are nutrients that the body needs to work properly. They boost the immune system, promote normal growth and development, and help cells regenerate.

Vitamins fall into two categories, fat soluble and water soluble. The fat-soluble vitamins, A, D, E, and K, dissolve in fat and can be stored in your body.

The water-soluble vitamins, C and the B-complex vitamins (such as vitamins B6, B12, niacin, riboflavin, and folate), need to dissolve in water before your body can absorb them.

Because of this, your body can't store these vitamins. Any vitamin C or B that your body doesn't use as it passes through your system, is lost especially through urination. So you need a fresh supply of these vitamins every day.

Your body needs larger amounts of some minerals, such as calcium, to grow and stay healthy. Other minerals like chromium, copper, iodine, iron, selenium, and zinc are called trace minerals because you only need very small amounts of them each day.

Vitamin deficiencies are common in the United States. The majority of people who should be taking vitamin and mineral supplements are people who are eating poor diets, pregnant women and senior citizens.

Before you take any other supplement, start with a moderately high-potency multi-vitamin. There are a lot of different types on the market.

High-potency supplements provide more value for your money, and some are formulated for men's health, women's health, diabetes, pregnancy, etc.

Most people typically start supplementing for one of the four reasons - they want a supplement that provides nutritional insurance against poor eating habits; they want to reduce their long-term risk of disease and disability; they'd like to reduce their risk of a specific disease that runs in their family; and they want to reduce symptoms of a health problem they already are dealing with, such as diabetes, heart disease, forgetfulness, or allergies.

Pediatricians may recommend a daily multi-vitamin or mineral supplement for:
- Kids who aren't eating regular, well-balanced meals made from fresh, whole foods
- Kids who are finicky eaters who simply aren't eating enough
- Kids with chronic medical conditions such as asthma or digestive problems
- Kids taking medications which can rob their bodies of nutrients and enzymes
- Kids who are active playing physically demanding sports
- Kids eating a lot of fast-food meals, convenience foods, and processed foods

- Kids on a vegetarian diet that might need an iron supplement
- Kids who drink a lot of carbonated sodas, which can leach vitamins and minerals from their bodies
- Kids on a dairy-free diet that might require them to take a calcium supplement or eat foods containing calcium
- Kids on other restricted diets

Whatever the reason, supplementing is a commitment. You should take your supplements consistently as part of a broader program (including good eating habits and regular physical activity) to prevent or reverse health problems.

How To Find the Right Supplements

Most minerals are bulkier than vitamins, and because of this, most supplements claiming to be a multi-vitamin/multi-mineral tend to scrimp on the minerals.

To avoid shortchanging yourself, consider taking a separate multi-mineral supplement. The supplement should also contain chromium, magnesium, potassium, selenium, zinc, and other important minerals.

Just because you have found the right supplement regimen to support your health today does not mean the same program will be ideal in 10 years.

Odds are, in 10 years, you will need more of some nutrients to offset age-related illnesses. You will have to modify your supplements, by type or dosage, if you are under more stress or change your exercise habits.

If you start taking a supplement to help with a specific health concern, apply the 30-day rule: If it doesn't seem to help within 30 days, stop taking it. If the symptoms then suddenly get worse, the supplement probably was helping, but the improvement was slow and hard to notice. Resume taking the supplement for another 30 days to find out.

Watch out for overlapping vitamins and minerals. If you're taking a multi-vitamin and want to add another formula, such as one to improve blood sugar, compare the ingredients. You may end up getting more of some vitamins or minerals than you need (though the excess is rarely harmful).

Take supplements at the right time. Most supplements should be taken with food. After all, supplements are nutrients and they usually work best with other nutrients. Take most supplements with breakfast or split them between breakfast and lunch.

You can take calcium supplements with magnesium throughout the day. Try to take calcium supplements at least 2 hours away from other supplements because they can strip other supplements of essential nutrients. It is important to take Vitamin D with your calcium supplements.

Where to Buy Vitamins and Minerals
Only buy vitamins from health food or whole food stores. Even though you can't find these stores as easily as grocery stores and other stores, they are essential to you renewing your health, so seek them out today.

To find local health food stores in your neighborhood, go to RenewLife.com and put your zip code in the store locator at the top. A list of all local health foods stores in your area should come up. The RenewLife.com products are popular and will probably be sold in these stores.

If you are buying vitamins from drug stores and other community stores (Walgreens, CVS, Wal-mart, Target, etc.), which are not whole or health food stores, chances are you are buying vitamins that contains *"dead chemicals,"* which means they were made in a lab and could be extremely harmful to your body.

Vitamin potency can be destroyed by antibiotics, consumption of alcohol and by sunlight so make sure that the container holding your vitamins is dark enough and keep vitamins and other supplements in a cool, dark place.

Be mindful of the expiration date on all vitamins and supplements, and discard them if you notice any change in odor or appearance.

The Immune System is Vital to Your Existence

As a kid many of us never got sick besides the normal childhood illnesses such as measles, mumps, and chicken pox. Back then our parents made sure we took castor oil, black draught laxative, and other natural remedies which boosted our immune systems.

But today because this generation no longer take these types of *"old folk remedies,"* the Standard American Diet (SAD), lack of exercise and sleep have all contributed to our bodies becoming more susceptible to diseases and illnesses causing us to have a weak immune system.

Everyone has either a weak or strong immune system. For those who have a weak system, it will be easier for them to catch illnesses than those with a strong immune system. If you have more than 2 colds a year, it's a good chance you might have a weak immune system.

Keeping the immune system functioning at its best is critical. When the system becomes weakened, it's unable to fight off invaders.

Anything from a cold to cancer or the development of autoimmune diseases can be the result of an immune system that is not functioning at its best.

The immune system gradually gets less effective as you age. It is a highly complex defense mechanism that helps us to fight infections. The immune system is our defense against invaders like germs, bacteria, viruses, yeast, fungus, and parasites.

Immune health and overall health go hand in hand. Eating right and taking the right supplements can help build a strong immune system.

Herbs, vitamins and minerals are powerful guardians and defenders of your health at a time when high-stress lifestyles and toxic environments take a toll on immune systems.

To keep a strong immune system you can:
- Eliminate toxic food and drink from your diet (eliminate junk food and a sugar-laden diet while eating simple meals in as natural state as possible)
- Detoxify your body often (colon, liver, kidneys)
- Strengthen your digestive/elimination system

- Get rid of personal care products containing toxic chemicals
- Get the toxins out of your home and workplace
- Add fresh, clean air to your environment whenever possible
- Keep your body well-mineralized
- Avoid taking excessive zinc and iron supplements
- Get a good night's sleep

Foods that improve the immune system include elderberry, button mushrooms, acai berry, oysters, watermelon, cabbage, almonds, grapefruit, garlic, spinach, tea, and broccoli.

CHAPTER 4
FASTING IS GOOD FOR YOU

What is Fasting?

For those of you who have been feeling sick, sluggish, or run-down or if you are suffering from some type of chronic or debilitating illness, you can heal your body sooner by fasting.

The *"common sense"* definition of fasting is the abstinence of food and substance, or a reduction in normal consumption. The dictionary definition is to keep from eating all or certain foods; to eat very little or nothing. This goes on around the clock for 24-hour periods.

The main reasons to fast is to lose weight; to grow spiritually; to enhance prayer; to cleanse the body; to purge the mind; to heal the body; and to recover from some debilitating state.

Other reasons to fast include:
- Fasting can remove unnecessary weight the natural way, plus learning how to keep it off for the rest of your life.
- Prolonged fasting can remove toxic waste dump now polluting the average adult's cells, tissues and organ storage areas such as chemical toxins, heavy metals, pesticides, drugs, intestinal parasites, etc.
- Fasting can help you regain the energy you use to have, perhaps when you were younger or more athletic.
- Fasting can elevate you out of a clouded consciousness, while heightening your mental clarity and all of your senses, allowing you to see

your life's options in a clearer perspective, and then act upon them wisely.
- Fasting can move you back toward your life's birthright potential of optimal health, increasing your happiness and healing power as you reset your body's odometer and greatly enhance your quality of life.

Fasting can help you heal with greater speed while cleansing your colon, liver, kidneys; purifying your blood; help you lose excess weight and water; flush out toxins; clear the eyes and tongue; and cleanse the breath.

Fasting is a safe and effective method of helping the body detoxify itself and move through the low cycle with greater speed and fewer symptoms. Every night when you sleep, you are fasting. When you are sick, you fast because most of the time you lose your appetite.

Fasting doesn't mean you totally starve yourself for days. What you need to understand is that overtime, toxins build up in your body as a result of the air you breathe, the water you drink and the food you eat.

These toxins continue to sink into your system causing a low and high cycle. During this time you will suffer from headaches, diarrhea, and even depression.

By fasting regularly you give your body time to rest but it's not just recommended in times of poor health.

How Long Should You Fast?

Depending on the length of the fast, it accomplishes different things such as a 3 day fast helps your body rid itself of toxins and cleanse the blood; A 5 day fast begins the process of healing and rebuilding the immune system; and a 10 day fast can take care of many problems before they arise and help to fight off illnesses including the degenerative diseases.

Fasting for a day or two probably won't hurt people who are generally healthy, provided they maintain an adequate fluid intake. However, fasting for long periods of time can be harmful.

Your body needs a variety of vitamins, minerals, and other nutrients from food to stay healthy. Not getting enough of these nutrients during fasting diets can lead to symptoms such as fatigue, dizziness, constipation, dehydration, gallstones, and cold intolerance. *Remember, it is possible to die if you fast too long!*

You can also try a slightly longer fast, or three days, which is good for those who have tried the one day fast and would like to extend it for a little bit longer. It's not a very challenging amount of time, but it is enough time to really give your body a good break from solid food.

A one day fast is not really enough time to draw toxins out of your body, but with a three day fast, the process of detoxification will begin. This means that you may actually feel bad during those three days, as your body expels toxins into the blood stream.

It's very important that you have bowel movements at least once a day, to ensure that your body is actually getting rid of those toxins properly.

It will also pay to do some skin brushing while on the juice fast, to ensure that your lymph system is assisting in the expulsion of toxins.

Whenever you fast for longer than three days, do so under the supervision of a doctor. Remember it takes years for the average body to wear down, therefore, it will take you some time to build it back up. So whenever you start to feel unwell, fast and feel better.

Why You Should Engage in Juicing

Juicing is the vital key to giving you a radiant, energetic life and truly optimal health. Not only will juicing fill you up but it will provide key nutrients that your body has probably been going without. However, it is important not to see juicing as a meal replacement, it is not. You still need to eat fresh, whole, organic vegetables and some fruit for fiber.

Certain precautions should be taken during fasts. First do not fast on water alone. An all-water fast releases toxins too quickly, causing headaches and worse. Instead follow a live juice diet which provides the body with vitamins, minerals and enzymes.

When fasting the first step should be to buy a good blender or juicer. I love the Vitamix Blender and Jack LaLanne Juicer. When you drink from a blender or juicer, the nutrients go straight into your system.

Juicing is a time-consuming process, so you'll probably be thinking to yourself, "I wonder if I can juice first thing and then drink it later?"

This isn't a great idea! Vegetable juice is very perishable so it's best to drink all of your juice immediately. However, if you're careful or use a more expensive juicer or blender, you can store it for up to 24 hours with only a moderate nutritional decline.

To prepare for a fast, eat only raw vegetables and fruits for two days. When on the fast, consume at least eight - 8 ounce glasses of distilled, pure/purified, or alkaline water a day, plus pure juices and cups of herbal tea.

Dilute all juices with water, adding about 1 part water to 3 parts juice. Do not drink orange or tomato juice, and avoid all juices made with sweeteners or other additives.

The best juice to use during a fast is fresh lemon juice. Add the juice of one lemon to a cup of warm water.

Fresh apple, beet, cabbage, carrot, celery, and grape juice are also good. Raw cabbage juice is especially good for ulcers, cancers and all colon problems. Just be sure to drink the cabbage juice as soon as it is prepared.

The best alkalizing juice is made up mostly of green vegetables and grasses. Green drinks which are made from green leafy vegetables are excellent detoxifiers. Green drinks are especially good for your body and have a rejuvenating effect.

These drinks can be made with alfalfa sprouts, cabbage, kale, dandelion greens, spinach, wheat grass and other green vegetables. Broccoli, celery, onions, parsley, radishes, rutabaga, and turnips should be used in small amounts only.

To sweeten and dilute green juices, try adding fresh carrot and apple juice. As a general rule, you should not combine fruit and vegetable juice. Apples are the only fruit that should be added to vegetable juice. The first meals after a fast should be frequent and small.

During a fast, as toxins are released from your body, you may experience the following symptoms: fatigue; body odor; dry, scaly skin; skin eruptions; headaches; dizziness; irritability; anxiety; confusion; nausea; coughing; diarrhea; dark urine; dark, foul smelling stools; body aches; insomnia; sinus and bronchial mucus discharge; and/or visual and hearing problems.

These symptoms are not serious and will pass. During a fast be sure to get plenty of rest including napping during the daytime.

Fasting will also improve longevity by delaying the onset of age-related diseases including Alzheimer's, heart disease, and diabetes.

<u>WARNINGS:</u>
- Even short-term fasting is not recommended for people with diabetes, because it can lead to dangerous dips and spikes in blood sugar.
- Women who are pregnant or breastfeeding, or anyone with a chronic disease, should not fast.
- If you are over 65, or if you need daily supplements, continue taking your vitamin and mineral supplements during the fast.

CHAPTER 5
STAY AWAY FROM MEAT

What You Really Need to Know About Eating Meat

Meat is animal flesh that is used as food. Most often, this means the skeletal muscle and associated fat. It may also describe other edible tissues such as organs, livers, skin, brains, bone marrow, kidneys, or lungs.

The goal is to cut down on the amount of meat you are eating and try to eat the right kind of meat such as Omega 3 meats (wild caught salmon, sardines, tuna, etc.). Try to be careful eating tuna over twice a week because of heavy metals.

When choosing meat, choose the leanest cuts of meat. If you have to eat meat, try to find a dependable butcher you can trust and choose choice cuts of meat.

People are under the assumption you need to eat meat to get protein and many think only protein can give them energy. This is not the case. As a matter of fact, some of the largest animals in the world eat a plant-based diet instead of meats such as the elephant and gorilla.

Being vegetarian does not mean your diet will be lacking in protein. Most plant foods contain protein and in fact it would be very difficult to design a vegetarian diet that is short on protein.

If you eat meat, it stays in your body for 3 days or longer turning into toxins and parasites. People who are *"meat-eaters"* especially *"heavy meat-eaters,"* might also be afflicted with parasites. Parasites come from "*undercooked*" pork and beef.

Parasites are common in people with chronic disease symptoms. It has been estimated that as many as 80% of ALL AMERICANS have intestinal parasites. A good intestinal cleanse from a health food store will also include a "parasite cleanse."

If you have parasites, the symptoms include nervousness; aches and pains that move from place to place in the body; mimicked appendicitis; ulcers and various digestive pain; nausea or diarrhea; itching; acne; foul breath; furred tongue; jaundice; fatigue; menstrual irregularities; and insomnia.

Red meat has been linked to heart disease. Sausage, bacon and hot dogs are linked to colorectal cancer. The goal is to eat meat in moderation only especially if you already have a problem with eating too much meat. Your daily intake of meat should be the size of a deck of cards.

Why You Should See the Food Inc. Movie

According to the Food Inc. Movie (FoodIncMovie.com) or food documentary, we can change the way food is grown in this country. We just need to spread the word to everyone we know to watch the movie. You can rent the movie, buy it off the website or from other outlets.

Some of the alarming facts revealed in the movie include:
• Four companies own and control all the meat in this country, which makes it easier for contamination and even harder for any oversight.

- The reason many cows get e-coli is because they are feed Genetically Modified corn instead of grass like years ago.

- Over 80% of beef in this country contains ammonia aka *"Mr. Clean."* This include meat for fast food and restaurant establishments and the school lunch program. Ammonia is used to try to remove the e-coli out of beef but it doesn't work. The equipment in slaughter houses is also cleaned with ammonia so this is another way that ammonia ends up in beef.

- Each hamburger you eat has the meat of at least 50 different cows. When they slaughter cows, it's impossible to clean them thoroughly especially after they have stood for days knee-deep in their own feces and the feces of at least 50 other cows, which have dried on their bodies. If just one of those cows has e-coli, then all their meat is contaminated.

- If you have to eat beef, stay away from frozen beef patties which stand a better chance of having e-coli. Instead go to a butcher and buy a shoulder, or cut beef out of your diet -- altogether.

- Over 70% of grocery carts contain fecal matter and e-coli. This comes from beef or the run-off (urine) of beef which gets on green foods located in fields next to where cows are located.

- According to CDC.gov, never buy a food that has been recalled more than once. Beef is recalled every 6 months in this country, so never buy or eat beef again.

- As of 2003, when USDA.gov went under DHS.gov, the USDA.gov only inspects 4% of the meat imported into this country so many times this meat might be contaminated with parasites.

Other movies you should buy and share with everyone you love besides the *"Food Inc. Movie"* include *Genetic Roulette; The World According to Monsanto; Forks Over Knives; Dirt: The Movie; Food Fight; Fresh; Killer at Large; King Corn; Super Size Me; The Garden; The Future of Food* (2004); *The Real Dirt on Farmer John; Food Stamped* – just to name a few.

How To Keep Down Inflammation in Your Body

Inflammation is the reaction of living tissue to injury or infection, characterized by heat, redness, swelling, and pain. Animal fat in the diet especially contains substances that are inflammatory. This is why you should cut down on how much meat you eat.

When dividing up meats, use different cutting boards for your meats and vegetables, so as not to contaminate your vegetables with drippings from your meats.

Mucus-producing foods such as eggs, chocolate, dairy products and fried foods also causes inflammation. So cut these foods out of your diet ASAP.

The Standard American Diet, ironically referred to as SAD, causes inflammation due to its excess levels of sugars, grains, and low levels of Omega-3 fatty acids.

Pain, anywhere in your body, can occur as part of inflammation. We know that long-lasting pain often comes with diseases that involve long-term inflammation. When you have chronic inflammation, your immune system is working overtime.

Too much inflammation can do the body harm, lead to immobility, weight loss, and a weakening of muscle tissue and the inability to fight disease.

Things that can trigger inflammation include drug overuse, exposure to environmental toxins, infections, injury, trauma, etc.

The pain of acute inflammation in your joints will grab your attention, but you probably won't notice the chronic inflammation in your vascular system, where it's doing damage every day.

This silent inflammation reduces your odds of a long life just as effectively as breathing an invisible, odorless poison gas. Chronic, low-level inflammation is now recognized to be a major part of every single degenerative disease from obesity to diabetes to cancer to Alzheimer's.

This kind of inflammation flies beneath the radar. It's happening right now in your body, but you're unaware of it.

Inflammatory chemicals are everywhere! Nearly everything that's an irritant to the system, the air pollution we breathe, the tobacco smoke we inhale directly or indirectly, the over 80,000 chemicals we're exposed to in our environment, have the potential to produce inflammation.

Inflammation is killing us! To extinguish the fire within us, you need to realize that a great deal of inflammation is under our control.

If you can put out the fire within, inflammation, or at least stop it from spreading, you'll be well ahead of the game when it comes to extending your life, as well as improving the quality of the years you have.

It is hardly coincidental that many of the healthful foods are found in the diets of the longest-lived people on the planet.

Some of the superstars of the food kingdoms when it comes to containing these natural anti-inflammatories include onions, garlic, and leeks; spices (ginger, turmeric, cinnamon, clover); leafy greens (spinach, kale, collard greens, chard); brassica vegetables (cabbage, brussels sprouts, cauliflower, broccoli); tomatoes; bell peppers; nuts and seeds; herbs (parsley, sage, rosemary, thyme, oregano, mint, tarragon, dill); tea (all types); flaxseeds and flax oil; etc.

CHAPTER 6
CHEW YOUR FOOD

The Correct Way to Eat Foods

The goal is to drink water (or lemon juice and water) 20 to 30 minutes before you eat, so you don't fill up on liquids when you eat.

This will help open up your digestive system and help food pass through your body. The body will then take what it needs as nutrients and enzymes and the rest will come out as waste.

Make sure you chew your food 30 to 60 times before swallowing, so it will turn into a liquid. You can then resume drinking liquids one hour after you eat.

Keep in mind when you don't chew your food, you are swallowing undigested food particles which can get stuck in the pores in your intestines especially meat and turn into toxins.

Some people choose to eat five or six small meals a day instead of three big meals, which will help anyone keep the weight off. However, remember don't go three and a half to four hours without eating something especially if you have hypoglycemia (low blood sugar).

Remember it takes 20 minutes for your stomach to tell your brain you are full, so eat slowly. Try to avoid watching T.V. or reading a book while you are eating so you can pay attention to how much you are eating and your chewing habits.

Is It Heartburn or Indigestion?

Many people have cured their indigestion (also acid reflex) by choosing to chew their food more slowly and not drinking liquids with their meals.

Indigestion is your body's way of telling you what you probably already know, that you ate too quickly or ate too much of the wrong foods. So listen to your body, make healthy food choices and don't scarf down your meals.

A greasy meal or a too-quick bite to eat, isn't worth the taste when it leaves you feeling uncomfortable long after the meal is finished.

Indigestion typically leads to one or more of the following symptoms: Feeling uncomfortably full or bloated just after you finish eating such as pain or burning in the stomach; frequent burping; an acidic taste in the mouth; excess gas; nausea or vomiting; diarrhea; or constipation.

Indigestion is particularly common in people who drink a lot of alcohol or caffeinated beverages; smoke; eat foods that are greasy and high in fat; eat very spicy foods; eat too quickly or eat too much food; eat while under stress; and have a history of heartburn.

Swallowing excess air while eating too quickly and exercising right after a big meal can also cause indigestion. Keep in mind that medications such as aspirin, ibuprofen, and certain antibiotics can cause an upset stomach.

CHAPTER 7
STOP EATING MUCUS-PRODUCING FOODS

We have become a culture of fast and easy, with no regard for healthy. Since the early fifties, when the fast food industry really took off, it made this jaded way of eating seem normal. The conditioning was so effective, that anyone who deviated was labeled a radical health nut.

But unless you buck the system and educate your own self, your health will eventually deteriorate and your energy will continue to drain out of your body.

If you are suffering from asthma, bad allergies and other illnesses that leave you congested in your sinuses and chest, it's a good chance you are also eating mucus-producing foods and have an acidic or toxic body.

The first thing you need to know upfront is that "*mucus-producing foods*" causes inflammation. These foods causes your body to swell on the inside and makes you very uncomfortable on the outside.

As we said earlier, these foods causes pain, sometimes excruciating pain, and who in their right mind want to be in pain? Some of the main foods that are mucus-producing are dairy products, eggs, chocolate, and fried foods.

Reasons You Should Avoid Dairy Products

Dairy products are a mucus-forming food so you need to be careful consuming any and all dairy products (milk, cheese, cottage cheese, yogurt, ice cream, etc.).

TEST YOURSELF! Stop eating all these mucus-producing foods especially dairy products for 2 to 3 weeks to see if you feel better.

You should have a major rise in energy. If you feel better after not consuming the foods, then cut them out of your diet completely! You don't need these foods. The goal is not to eat anything that is "altered." Dairy products are altered!

Other reasons to avoid milk:
- **Milk often contains unwanted ingredients:** Under current industrial methods, cow's milk is often a toxic bovine brew of man-made ingredients like bio-engineered hormones, antibiotics (55% of U.S. antibiotics are fed to livestock), and pesticides, all of which are bad for us and the environment. For example, drugs pumped into livestock often re-visit us in our water supply.

- **Cow's milk is for cows:** The biochemical make-up of cow's milk is perfectly suited to turn a 65-pound newborn calf into a 400-pound cow in one year. So some may like cow's milk but drinking it is both unnecessary and potentially harmful.

- **Milk makes you fat:** According to leading experts, three glasses of low-fat milk add more than 300 calories a day. This is a real issue for the millions of Americans who are trying to control their weight.

- **Milk is actually a poor source for dietary calcium:** Humans, like cows, gorillas and elephants, can get all the calcium they need from a plant-based diet.

What's more, millions of Americans are lactose intolerance, especially African Americans, and even small amounts of milk give them stomach aches, gas, or other problems. This means they are allergic to dairy products and need to cut it out of their diets, as soon as possible.

How To Get Calcium for Strong Bones

When it comes to bone health, it's particularly important to avoid what we call the "bone robbers." If you want good bones, you have to limit your alcohol intake; stop smoking; don't salt your food excessively; go easy on the sugar; and don't commune soda.

Contrary to popular belief, milk may increase the likelihood of osteoporosis. It is still widely accepted that the calcium in dairy products will strengthen our bones and help prevent osteoporosis, but studies show that foods originating from animal sources (like milk) make the blood acidic.

When this occurs, the blood leeches calcium from the bones to increase alkalinity. While this works wonders for the pH balance of your blood, it sets your calcium-depleted bones up for osteoporosis.

Salt is a major culprit that is depriving the body of calcium. The more salt you eat, the more calcium gets carried away by urine. Sticking to low-salt diets can help you keep more calcium to strengthen your bones. If you have high blood pressure avoid salt all together!

Calcium just doesn't come from dairy products. Calcium is plentiful in certain vegetables. A half a cup of Chinese cabbage provides calcium equal to that in a 8 ounce glass of milk. One cup of turnip greens offers 200 mg of calcium. Spinach and broccoli contains some calcium.

Also salmon and other types of fatty fish offer an array of bone-boosting nutrients, which contains calcium as well as vitamin D, which assist in calcium absorption.

Eating 3 ounces of canned sardines delivers a little more calcium than a cup of milk. Nuts such as almonds, pistachios and sunflower seeds are high in calcium and can boost bone health in several ways.

Dairy products and meat promotes hot flashes in women and contributes to a loss of calcium from the bones. Remember everyone especially women need calcium especially for their bones as they age.

In place of milk, you can take a calcium supplement with magnesium and vitamin D. Magnesium helps with constipation.

Eating dairy products and meats are the main reasons you need to detoxify your body regularly. So give yourself a break, if you don't want to engage in regular detoxification programs, cut milk and meat from your diet. Remember the goal is *"bad stuff out and good stuff in."*

Why You Should Avoid Processed Foods

Processed foods are considered to be bad foods or non-foods. Processed foods are the reason people are overweight and feel tired, sluggish and run-down.

Processed foods are found in a can, box, jar, package or some other wrapping or container. At least 90% of processed foods at grocery stores contain Genetically Modified (GM) foods.

If you eat processed foods you are giving yourself empty calories, not nutrients because the foods have been altered from their original state.

Food processing typically takes harvested crops or butchered animal products and uses these to produce marketable and often long shelf-life food products.

These foods are foods that can impair the immune system such as artificial sweeteners, carbonated soft drinks, chocolate, eggs, fried foods, junk foods, pork, red meat, sugar, white flour products, foods containing preservatives or heavy spices, and chips and similar snack foods.

If you are a product of a large family who always struggled to keep food on the table, then getting healthier might be more of a challenge for you especially if you were expected to eat whatever your parents fed you.

Back then processed and refined foods were the mainstay diet in most American households. But now there must be a new level of thinking especially with over 90% of foods in neighborhood grocery stores containing components or derivatives of Genetically Modified foods.

Because of what they have placed in processed foods (transfat, high fructose corn syrup, GMOs, etc.), over the past 20 years, you must now think outside the box.

Why You Should Avoid Canned Foods
Canned foods which are also processed foods are definitely associated with the obesity problem in this country.

Do not use canned vegetables or boxed vegetable dishes, because they usually contain significant amounts of salt and other unhealthy additives. Salt is added to canned foods and other processed foods in order for the food to have a longer shelf-life.

Canned foods or foods that you buy in a can, also have BPA poisoning in their lining. What most people are unaware of is that BPA is still widely used in the food industry.

If you consume anything in a can or anything in polycarbonate plastic containers (not labeled as BPA-free), or if you regularly microwave those plastic containers, put them in the dishwasher at high temperatures, or put hot foods directly into them after cooking, you are being exposed to BPA.

If you have a baby that you are formula feeding, you are likely exposing your child to BPA through the formula itself, which is almost assuredly packaged in a BPA-lined can.

When preparing foods, use only glass, stainless steel, or iron pots and pans. Foods cooked or stored in aluminum is harmful, so don't use this cookware or utensils.

When this food is consumed, the aluminum is absorbed by the body, where it accumulates in the brain and nervous system tissues.

6 Harmful Ingredients to Always Avoid
Read food labels and always avoid sugar; high fructose corn syrup; red and yellow dye; enriched white bread; transfat (found in processed foods); and saturated fat (found in meats).

Sugar: There may be hidden sugars hiding in your cabinets and pantries. You can eliminate them by throwing away any foods that contains high amounts of added sugars.

This includes everything from tomato sauces to ketchup to peanut butter. Be especially wary of low-fat items as they often contain more sugar to make them taste better.

When purging your kitchen, be on the lookout for names such as fructose, maltose, sorbitol, evaporated cane juice, syrups, xylitol, sugars ending in "ol" or "ose." Instead of sugar, try using an alternative sweetener stevia or chicory from health food stores.

Another reason not to eat sugar or not to allow your kids to eat it, is that sugar retards growth and refined sugars turns off the brain. In other words, giving your kids sugar causes a lack of growth and lack of brain function. Is that what you want for your children or family?

Excessive amounts of sugar can cause gallstones to form so obesity and gallbladder disease are related. Gallstones run in families, and women are twice as likely to form gallstones as men. A detoxification program for the liver and colon is important for improved gallbladder function.

Though fruits have many good vitamins and minerals and is rich in fiber, fruits are also filled with sugar. Despite what some nutritionists claim, there is no difference in your body between natural sugars and any other kind. Sugar is sugar, it doesn't matter!

With the exception of lemons, limes, and occasionally non-sweet grapefruits, fruits must be avoided to gain a healthy balanced body. You can get all the same nutritional benefits from fresh, raw, green organic vegetables, without the negative side effects.

High Fructose Corn Syrup: In the old days, manufacturers were highly motivated to find a solution to the problem of expensive sugar, which was the creation of *"high-fructose corn syrup."* High-fructose corn syrup really isn't that different from table sugar.

High-fructose corn syrup, at least the most common kind, the kind in soft drinks, is 55 percent fructose and 45 percent glucose. It's not a huge difference from the 50/50 mix in plain old sugar. The problem is, it's everywhere!

The low-cost of high-fructose corn syrup allowed the explosion of 20-ounce sodas, Sugar Big Gulps, and an explosion of candies, bakery items, and ice cream novelties that would have been just too costly if they were all made with sugar.

Red & Yellow Dye: Many people are allergic to food colorings. Read labels carefully! If you are allergic to red and yellow food dye, try to avoid any food products that contain artificial color. Other food additives to avoid include vanilla, benzaldehyde, eucalyptol, monosodium glutamate (MSG), BHT-BHA, benzoates and annatto.

Red and yellow food dye coloring is everywhere there are sweets. Many cakes, pies, and candies contain this harmful ingredient which is linked to ADHD, cancer, allergies, etc.

Enriched White Bread: When commercially prepared white bread first became widely available during the early twentieth century, it was discovered that it was not very nutritious.

Most of the important nutrients in the wheat were eliminated when producing white flour, resulting in white bread that was also lacking in nutrients.

It was determined that people who relied heavily on foods made from processed white flour and cornmeal were becoming ill due to a lack of B vitamins. White bread contains very little fiber, which is important for digestive health.

Even though bread will fill you up quicker, it has no nutritional value, and will turn acidic (or into sugar), along with other white foods in your body.

So avoid any white food (flour, bread, pasta, potatoes, rice, etc.). These foods alone is a major reason for the explosion of diabetes in this country. Read my article *"Diabetes 101: The Number One Killer of African Americans."*

<u>Transfat (found in processed foods):</u> Transfat is found mainly in deep-fried fast foods and processed foods made with margarine or shortening. It's created by a process called hydrogenation, that's used by food manufacturers to improve the stability of vegetable oils and to convert liquid oils into solid fats to get the right consistency in foods such as cakes and pastries.

Transfats are also added in processed foods to give it a longer shelf life. So read labels and cut out this ingredient which is extremely bad for you. Look for food labels that reads "0" Transfat.

<u>Saturated Fats (found in meats):</u> Look for food labels that reads "0" Saturated Fats. Many saturated fats are found in meats. Eating foods that contain saturated fats raises the level of cholesterol in your blood. High levels of blood cholesterol increase your risk of heart disease and stroke.

Pay Attention to Your Allergies

There are two types of allergies, "*Food*" and "*Environmental*" allergies which cause people to suffer needlessly. Environmental allergies are also called "airborne" allergies. Both types of allergies can cause you to be tired; miss days at work; have a chronic sore throat; feel achy; and can affect all parts of your body.

Food Allergies
Many processed foods causes "food allergies" and "food sensitivities" that can place stress on the immune system, so try to figure out which foods you need to eliminate from your diet.

If your allergies are thought to be "food related," keep a food diary and track foods eaten and the body's response to them in order to identify offending foods.

Some of the foods that you can be allergic to include -- milk or dairy products, eggs, nuts, avocadoes, rice, wheat, soy, corn, grapes, strawberries, cantaloupes, chocolate, peanuts, fish, shellfish, etc.

Remember Genetically Modified foods causes food allergies. Food allergies causes depression. If you are eating GMOs, more than likely your body will have some type of allergic reaction to most of these foods.

It doesn't mean you will break out in red spots, but more than likely, these foods will cause you to feel sluggish or run-down. Food should give you energy, not make you feel tired or exhausted.

My holistic doctor who is also a chiropractor told me I was allergic to oatmeal, strawberries, MSG, food additives, coffee and aluminum.

Once I stopped eating these foods or foods that contained the ingredients, I started feeling absolutely great! My advice to anyone is, don't wait another moment, get tested today from a holistic specialist or chiropractor who specializes in this field.

Food allergies can mask themselves in different ways including acne, especially pimples on the chin or around the mouth; epilepsy; arthritis; asthma; chest and shoulder pain; colitis; depression; fatigue; food cravings; headaches; hemorrhoids; insomnia; intestinal problems; muscle disorder; obesity; sinus problems; ulcers and unexplained dramatic weight gain or loss.

Food allergies often cause symptoms that mimic bladder infections. Food allergies are linked to hypoglycemia.

Environmental Allergies
People might have an environmental allergy to ragweed, mold, oak, cockroaches, dust mikes, feathers, horses, weeds, trees, pollen, the urine and saliva of a dog, etc.

For environmental or airborne allergies, you can purchase an air filter to clean pollen, mold, and dust from your home or office.

Frequent exposure to allergens combined with a weakened immune system can result in the development of allergies. If you can avoid contact with known allergens, you can reduce the misery of allergy symptoms.

Some hay fever sufferers experience relief almost as soon as they drink two or more glasses of water. The best time to take allergy or asthma medication is between 6:00 and 8:00 a.m.

Pollen season can play havoc on allergy sufferers. If you suffer from seasonal allergies you should:
- Keep windows closed in your home and car
- Buy special home or car filters
- Use the recirculate setting on your car air conditioner
- Use your home air conditioner to deliver clean, dry, and cool air
- Do not use an attic fan for ventilation
- Exercise indoors when possible
- Schedule outdoor activities carefully (pollen counts are highest early in the morning so outdoor activities/exercises in the evening are best)
- Avoid outdoors on dry windy days
- Take a vacation during the pollen season (Seashore is likely to have lower pollen exposures)
- Avoid mowing lawns, raking or blowing leaves, it stirs up pollens and molds
- Wash your clothes and your hair after being out in the pollen
- Don't hang your sheets and clothes out to dry in the pollen
- Wash your pet after being out in the pollen
- Use over-the-counter antihistamines

CHAPTER 8
CONSTANTLY EXPEL TOXINS FROM YOUR BODY

Remember we live in an imperfect world so toxins are constantly coming into our bodies through the food we eat, water we drink and air we breathe.

Toxins are a poisonous substance, especially one produced by a living organism. Toxins must be broken down or excreted from your body before building up to dangerous levels.

Ways to Expel Toxins from Your Body

Since most people have too many toxins coming in, and not enough going out, the goal is to keep the toxins exiting your body.

Three ways to expel or keep these toxins exiting your body include sweating through your skin (in a sitz bath, exercising, sauna or steam room); through your urine (regular fasting and detoxing); and through your waste (regular fasting and detoxing).

The skin is actually referred to as "*the third kidney.*" One of the best ways to sweat toxins out of your body include -- engaging in some type of cardiovascular exercise (fast or power walking, running, aerobics, swimming, bicycling/spinning, etc.).

You can also sweat toxins out of your body by joining a gym and sweating in a sauna or steam room. Sitting in the sauna increases blood circulation, burn calories, lowers blood pressure and removes toxins.

Hot and Cold Sitz Baths

As a form of hydrotherapy, the use of hot and cold water has been used to restore and maintain health. The sitz bath increases blood flow to the pelvic and abdominal areas, and thus can help reduce inflammation and otherwise alleviate a variety of problems.

Each bath can be helpful in different ways:
1. _Hot sitz baths_ are particularly helpful for such disorders as hemorrhoids, muscular disorders, painful ovaries and testicles, prostate problems, and uterine cramps.
2. _Cold sitz baths_ are helpful in the treatment of constipation, impotence, inflammation, muscle disorders, and vaginal discharge.

Alternating hot and cold sitz baths can help relieve abdominal disorders, congestion, foot infections, headaches, muscle disorders and swollen ankles.

To prepare a sitz bath, put in a cup of epsom salt or baking soda (use aluminum free from health food stores). Fill a tub or basin so that the water covers the hips and reaches the middle of the abdomen.

If possible, place the water in a tub or basin that will allow you to immerse just the pelvis and abdominal regions. You may wish to cover your body with a sheet or blanket to increase your comfort. Stay in the bath from 20 - 40 minutes.

Get out of the tub slowly, allowing the water to drain from the tub. Dry yourself, and rest or cool down five to ten minutes until you are no longer perspiring. Keep yourself warm and comfortable and covered.

Detoxification Process and Sitz Baths
While you are engaged in a detoxification program of your colon, liver, or kidneys or during the fasting process, it will be extremely important for you to assist the toxins to exit your body.

The steps in this chapter especially need to go hand-in-hand with the fasting or the detoxification process.

You might not feel like going to a gym and sweating in the sauna or steam room while you are fasting or detoxifying your body, but you might feel like engaging in a sitz bath at home.

Remember your lifestyle is mainly up to you. The quicker the toxins exit your body and you create new habits that will cut down on the amount of toxins in your food, water and environment, the sooner you will start feeling like your old energetic self again.

CHAPTER 9
DRINK THE RIGHT TYPE OF WATER

Many people are confused as to how much water they should drink. How much water do you need every day? Drink at least 1 liter (4 cups equals one liter) of water a day for every 30 pounds of body weight.

So figure out how much water you should drink everyday. Don't count sodas, coffee, milk, juices, teas, and any other beverages.

What is the Right Type of Water?

Many people are unsure of what type of water to drink. The wrong type of water can make you sick, tired, and fat.

You should ONLY drink distilled, pure/purified or alkaline water. You can put pH drops from health food stores in distilled or pure/purified water to make it more alkaline.

Alkaline water is the best water to drink. It is sold in health and whole foods stores. Getting liberal amounts of alkaline water (having a pH between 9 and 11), which neutralizes stored acid wastes and, if consumed every day in conjunction with a good diet, gently removes the acids from the body.

Other top reasons to drink Alkaline Water include:
- It's a powerful antioxidant that helps scavenge free radicals in the body.
- Alkalizing increases the body's natural defenses and strengthens immunity.
- Alkaline water cleanses and detoxifies the body.
- Alkaline water provides super-hydration for all of

the body's cells.
- Alkaline water brings the body back into balance by slowing down the aging process; Promoting healthy weight loss; Boosting immunity; and increasing absorption of minerals and vitamins.

Other types of water will make you dehydrated and if your body is dehydrated, it will not do what it is supposed to do.

Once you change the type of water that you are drinking, it can take as little as three days for you to feel a difference. Your body will feel cooler and you will feel better.

If you have an extremely toxic or acidic body, it means your pH balance is off. Remember the goal is to have an alkaline body.

It will most likely be quite challenging to rehydrate your body, but don't get discouraged. You should start feeling better over the next few days or weeks.

If you have a weight problem, your food cravings may be a sign of thirst, not hunger! Always drink room temperature water because cold water and drinks interferes with your digestive process.

Drinking water at the correct time maximizes its effectiveness on the human body. You should drink water every hour.

Never drink water with your meals. Instead drink water 20 or 30 minutes before each meal. Then resume your water intake one hour after your meals.

Causes of Dehydration

Over 75% of people are chronically dehydrated. Pay attention to your body. If you crave salt, it's a good chance you are dehydrated.

Dehydration is a condition that occurs when the loss of body fluids, mostly water, exceeds the amount that is taken in.

We lose water every day in the form of water vapor in the breath we exhale and as water in our sweat, urine, and stool.

Along with the water, small amounts of salts are also lost. When we lose too much water, our bodies may become out of balance or dehydrated. *Just remember severe dehydration can lead to death!*

Many conditions may cause rapid and continued fluid losses and lead to dehydration such as fever, heat exposure, and too much exercise; vomiting, diarrhea, and increased urination due to infection; diseases such as diabetes; the inability to seek appropriate water and food (an infant or disabled person, for example); an impaired ability to drink (someone in a coma or on a respirator or a sick infant who cannot suck on a bottle are common examples); no access to safe drinking water; and significant injuries to skin, such as burns or mouth sores, or severe skin diseases or infections (water is lost through the damaged skin).

Learn more about how women lose their hair because of dehydration and other reasons in my book *"My Hair, My Crown, My Glory: A Woman's Guide to Growing Gorgeous Hair"* at http://www.AngelsPress.com.

Stop Drinking Tap Water

Many people assume that when they turn on the kitchen tap, they are getting clean, safe, healthy drinking water. Unfortunately, this often is not the case. Tap water is full of harmful chemicals that the body cannot use.

If you have to drink or use tap water, never use the first water drawn from your tap. Let it run for at least three minutes before you use it. Never boil water longer than necessary, five minutes is enough.

Some of the undesirable substances found in water include radon, fluoride, arsenic, iron, lead, copper and other heavy metals. Others include fertilizers, asbestos, cyanides, herbicides, pesticides, and industrial chemicals, which may leach into ground water through the soil or into tap water from plumbing pipes.

According to the Centers for Disease Control and Prevention (CDC.gov), almost 1,000,000 people in the U.S. get sick every year from contaminated water, and many will die from waterborne diseases.

For people who live in rural areas, well water is extremely bad for you. Having a filter on your kitchen sink or refrigerator will not make a difference. Many of these filters are not any good.

Many of these chemicals have been linked to cancer and many other disorders. Because of concerns over the safety and health effects of tap water, many people today are turning to bottled water.

While the EPA.gov is charged with the regulation of public water supplies, it is the FDA.gov that has responsibility for overseeing the quality and safety of bottled drinking water.

Drink Water First Thing in the Morning
Start the morning with eight ounces of water and the juice of an organic lemon. Even better make sure the water is warm. This step will activate your liver and you will be able to feel the energy right away.

Always try to use organic lemons. If you don't have any organic or plain lemons to put in your water, drink water anyway. It will open up your digestive system and allow food to pass through your system.

Never, ever skip breakfast. It's the most important meal of the day. Make sure you eat small meals every three and a half to four hours (5 or 6 times a day) instead of three large meals a day.

Always keep a glass or bottle of water by your bed at night. If you have trouble sleeping, instead of eating something, drink a glass of water instead.

Going into the kitchen for water or a snack will do nothing but wake you out of your sound sleep and put weight on you especially if you are already overweight.

You know you are drinking enough water when you can place a piece of newspaper in your toilet and can read the words through your urine.

To kill odor from your urine buy natural cranberry juice from a health food store.

CHAPTER 10
STOP TAKING PHARMACEUTICALS

Long Term Effects of Medications

The pharmaceutical industry in this country will always be "**BIG BUSINESS.**" In other words, their only goals are to keep you on medications.

I discovered that doctors are programmed and conditioned by the pharmaceutical industry and they will not answer your questions because they don't know the answers. The goal is to get a doctor who is an outside-the-box thinker.

Antibiotic overuse has become a pandemic problem. They are used in animal feed to make animals grow more quickly and they are handed out like candy by many doctors to people with almost any ailment.

Even antidepressants are handed out to people suffering from just about any type of ailment. OB/GYN doctors are handing out antidepressants to women who have postpartum depression or baby blues.

Some women have more severe symptoms of the baby blues or symptoms that last longer than a few days. This is postpartum depression.

Postpartum depression is an illness, like diabetes or heart disease. But no one should ever be given *"mind-altering"* medications like antidepressants unless they are monitored by the mental health community (psychiatrists, psychologists, mental health therapists, etc.).

Many people need to understand the long term effect of medications. Medications, over-the-counter (OTC) or prescribed, can ravage your internal organs and eventually cause them to give out especially your liver which detoxifies these medications.

There is a good chance that pharmaceutical use over the years has contributed to your organs becoming clogged, turning hard and slowing you down. So give your organs a break and get off all medications as soon as possible.

The goal is to reverse any damage that these pharmaceuticals have caused before it's too late. When one organ fails, they all fail because your organs work as a team.

In many communities, especially in African American communities, they do not donate organs, so it's extremely important to hang onto the organs that you already have.

The goal is to slowly take yourself off all medications. Chances are your unhealthy eating habits probably contributed to the reasons you were taking the pharmaceuticals in the first place.

The pharmaceuticals simply acted as a band-aid which covered up the real reason you had the problem.

Health Food Stores vs. Drug Stores
Health Food Stores: To find health food stores in your neighborhood, go to RenewLife.com and put your zip code in the store locator at the top of the page.

The goal is to find a health food store or two with a line of natural detoxification products for your colon, liver, and kidneys, vitamin and mineral supplements, and other natural products (toothpaste, soaps, deodorants, natural hair, skin and nail products, sunscreen, sea salt, alkaline water, etc.).

Many remedies that work from health food stores are natural. One of the natural remedies is known as "homeopathic remedies," which work very well. Homeopathy is a complete system of healing discovered 200 years ago.

It has its own method of diagnosing and its own special remedies. The remedies have no harmful side effects (like most medications) and are not addictive (like some medications).

They are safe for adults, the elderly, and for babies and children. Even pregnant women can take homeopathic remedies safely.

Drug Stores: Over-the-counter (OTC) drugs at drugstores are medicines that may be sold directly to a consumer without a prescription from a health care professional. Prescription drugs may only be sold to consumers possessing a valid prescription.

Millions of people take non-prescription or over-the-counter (OTC) medications. Taking over-the-counter medications incorrectly can trigger dizzy spells, jitters and gastrointestinal distress and eventually lead to ulcers and other health concerns.

Many of these medicines contain the same active ingredient even if they're marketed to treat different symptoms, so it is easy to double up unknowingly. Also combination formulas can contain drugs you don't need.

OTC and prescription medications might cause side effects. A side effect is usually regarded as an undesirable secondary effect which occurs in addition to the desired therapeutic effect of a drug or medication.

Side effects may vary for each individual depending on the person's disease state, age, weight, gender, ethnicity and general health.

Be proactive when taking any medications especially prescribed medications. Medical mistakes are made because there are over 1400 drugs that sound alike; people mix up medications; people take the wrong doses; people take medications with wrong foods; and people mix herbal supplements with medications.

That's why it's is extremely important to provide your doctor with a list of all the medications (other prescriptions, over-the-counter medications, herbal supplements, etc.) you are taking before he/she prescribes you any type of medication.

The side effects should be listed with the prescriptions but always talk to the doctor that prescribed the medication about any potential side effects.

You can also ask the pharmacist that filled the prescription and even go to WEBMD.com and look up potential side effects for any and all medications.

Side effects can occur when commencing, decreasing/increasing dosages, or ending a drug or medication regimen.

When side effects of a drug or medication are severe, the dosage may be adjusted or a second medication may be prescribed. Lifestyle or dietary changes may also help to minimize side effects.

What the New Healthcare Reform Bill Means For You

1. ***Kids With Health Problems:*** The new healthcare reform legislation prohibits insurers from excluding from coverage children with pre-existing health conditions. This provision takes effect immediately. The bill would also prohibit insurers from excluding adults with pre-existing conditions, but not until 2014.

2. ***Older Children and Parental Insurance:*** Dependent children up to age 26 will be able to stay on their parent's family policy (There's no special regulation as to what this will cost, however). Currently, states regulate the age at which children are kicked off their parents' insurance policies. Generally, it's around 18 years old.

3. ***Children's Health Insurance Program:*** Kid's eligibility for the popular CHIP (Children's Health Insurance Program), which helps lower-income families, must be maintained under the bill. States, even if hard-pressed by budget shortfalls, will not be able to cut children from the program until 2019.

4. ***Wellness Program:*** Under bill language, qualified health plans will have to provide with no cost-sharing immunizations and other preventive health services for infants, children, and adolescents.

5. ***Tax Penalty:*** Starting in 2014, all Americans (and people from other countries who are in the U.S. legally) must have a minimum level of health insurance coverage. If they don't, they'll pay a tax penalty. The penalty starts out small in 2014, but it will get bigger

over time. To avoid the penalty, you'll need to show on your tax return that you have some type of health coverage.

What To Do If You Don't Have Health Insurance
If you lose your health insurance or if you don't have health insurance be proactive by asking your doctor's office about a payment plan; ask for generic drugs; ask for samples from doctors; know your rights; appeal any claim; and commit to your recovery by empowering yourself.

For people who don't have health insurance, there are free clinics throughout their communities. Most community clinics provide low-cost medicine under the same roof or at nearby pharmacies.

Pharmaceutical Research and Manufacturers of America, the drug makers' trade group, provides free and low-cost drugs through its Partnership for Prescription Assistance (PPARX.org). Individual drug makers often have their own programs that offer free or reduced-cost drugs as well.

Community health centers, partially funded by the federal government, provide uninsured Americans with a regular doctor who knows their health situations and can help them manage chronic diseases.

The clinics offer treatment according to the patient's ability to pay and in some cases, for free. The closest of the 1,250 centers can be located at www.findahealthcenter.hrsa.gov.

How To Limit Trips to Emergency Rooms (ER)
The key to staying healthy and avoiding trips to emergency rooms (ER) are to have a primary physician

and go in for regular office visits. However, if you have an urgent problem, don't skip the emergency room.

Hospitals are often willing to make a payment plan and may even write off some of your bill. But the patient has to take the first step.

When the emergency is over, contacting the billing department as soon as possible will give you the best chance to reduce your costs. Once it gets turned over to a collection agency, the chances for charity basically go away.

Negotiating with the hospital is exactly what the insurance companies do. Insurers may pay only $3,000 for a procedure that a hospital will routinely bill an uninsured individual $9,000. Patients should ask that they be given the same rate as the insurers.

The billing department will tell you initially that you have to pay the full amount. Ask to speak to a supervisor. Keep notes of these conversations. Be polite and persistent!

Pick a Board Certified Doctor

When selecting a doctor, chose one that is *"board certified."* Many people recommend asking your doctor questions about their qualifications, including whether or not he or she is board certified. But what exactly does that mean?

The American Board of Medical Specialties (ABMS) is recognized as the "gold standards" in physician's certifications.

Certification by an ABMS Member Board involves a rigorous process of testing, peer evaluations and periodic recertification that is designed and administered by specialists in the specific area of medicine. Being board certified simply means better care for patients.

Don't Be Afraid to Switch Doctors
Many people are not comfortable with their doctors, therefore, they should find a doctor that they feel comfortable with. If you can't afford needed medications or if you lose your health insurance, start by talking to your doctor.

Tell your doctor about your change in status and ask if there is any flexibility on fees. Many physicians will offer a sliding scale or reduced payments to maintain the relationship.

He or she may be able to help with samples or in finding programs to get you what you need. When or if something does go wrong, you want to go to someone who you have a relationship with or someone who already knows your medical history.

If you are diagnosed with an illness, be proactive and get "*second*" and "*third*" opinions. If you are told you have an illness or disease where biopsies are taken and there are extra specimens, you can take your specimens with you to get another opinion, so ask for these specimens.

Find a High-Tech Hospital
Many hospitals are using a 19th century tool, a pen, in the 21st century. Bar coding has reduced error rates to "0 percent" so it's important to select a hospital that is high tech for you and your family members.

Many mistakes occur at hospitals all the time. One of the main reasons for mistakes in hospitals is nurses who are working 24-hour shifts.

Other mistakes that occur include over 14,000 patients report waking up during surgeries; many have reported that doctors operated on wrong body parts (breast); doctors have also operated on the wrong side of the brain; others have reported that doctors have left surgical equipment in patients such as sponges or scissors (this occurs at least 40 times a week in the U.S.), etc.

To avoid errors in hospitals pick a high-tech hospital; find a hospital with a checklist; make friends with your "hospitalist" (a specialist in inpatient medicine that can help you get procedures and get out of the hospital); avoid chit chat with doctors; if you are scheduled for surgery, mark your body (aka *"here"* and *"not here"*); know what medicines you are taking and carry them with you; be a smart patient (be brave enough to speak up or stand up not just for yourself but for the guy behind you).

To keep down catching germs in hospitals insist that doctors wash their hands and clean their stereoscopes; use hand sanitizer and insist that your visitors use it also; don't let anyone bring flowers or plants (they might contain a fungi and it's never a good idea to sleep in a room with flowers and plants); don't let anyone sit on your bed; and always clean television remotes.

Make sure you have a "hospital advocate" who should be a family member or friend who can keep up with the checklist, all your medications and talk to the doctors.

If a family member will be in the hospital for a while, this advocate should make a list of family members, friends or think about hiring healthcare aids and workers to sit with them in the daytime and at night especially if the patients are elderly.

Many elderly people need people to sit with them during the day and at night. They can get out of bed and slip and fall.

Most people especially the elderly, who break their hips, die within 2 years due to a sedentary lifestyle. The hospital also might have a list of healthcare aids and workers, so ask for it.

The goal is to get out of the hospital as soon as possible. Many people catch staph and other infections as long as they remain in hospitals.

People who stay there with them also get infections from hospitals so the goal is to recuperate at home in a clean and sterile environment.

Know Your Numbers and Save Your Life

We are all obsessed with numbers in our lives, our age, our weight, our height, etc. But there are some numbers that can literally save your life, but only if you know what they are and understand what they really mean.

A *"Lipid Panel"* or *"Lipid Profile"* with a 12 hour fast is needed to obtain the correct numbers for your cholesterol, blood glucose (blood sugar) and triglyceride level.

Adults 20 years old and older should get a lipid profile every five years. Most people up to the age of 40 can go to the doctor once a year for a physical if there is no underlining health issues or if they do not have family histories of diseases.

Others especially those 50 and over should have a complete physical examination every 6 months by their doctors in order to keep their numbers in range. Doctor's visits every 3 months are needed if there are underlining health issues and family histories of diseases.

No matter your age, if you have some type of underlining health issue and are taking medications, you should visit your doctor at least every 3 months to make sure your numbers stay in range.

Some of the numbers you need to be aware of include:
Cholesterol: Abnormal cholesterol levels such as high LDL (bad cholesterol) or low HDL (good cholesterol) are a major risk factor for heart disease and stroke. You should get this number checked regularly by age 40 (earlier if you have diabetes, high blood pressure, family history of heart disease, or you smoke).

If your doctor tells you that your cholesterol levels are out of range, it is essential that you avoid smoking, eat a healthy diet, and get regular exercise and plenty of rest while keeping your weight in check.

The numbers for your cholesterol should be:
- **Total blood (serum) cholesterol level:** Less than 200 mg/dL is considered desirable; 200 to 239 mg/dL is considered borderline-high risk; 240 mg/dL and over is a high risk to your health.

- **HDL cholesterol level:** Less than 40 mg/dL for men or less than 50 mg/dL for women means a higher risk for heart disease; For men, 40 to 50 mg/dL is considered average; For women, 50 to 60 mg/dL is considered average.

- **LDL cholesterol level:** Less than 100 mg/dL is optimal; 100 to 129 mg/dL is near or above optimal; 130 to 159 mg/dL is considered borderline high; 160 to 189 mg/dL is high; 190 mg/dL and above is considered to be very high.

<u>Blood Glucose (Blood Sugar):</u> Low blood sugar is *hypoglycemia* and high blood sugar is *diabetes*. You should have your blood glucose checked every year starting at age 45 or earlier, earlier or more often if you have family history or underlining health issues. Your glucose level should be less than 100. If it is 125, then you have pre-diabetes.

<u>High Blood Pressure aka Hypertension:</u> You should have your blood pressure checked every year. Most of the time your blood pressure is checked when you visit the doctor. Your blood pressure or hypertension level should be less than 120/80.

An ideal blood pressure is 115/75. If the level is 140/90 or higher then you have high blood pressure and should be on medications to bring the number down. If your numbers are 130/80, then this is high if you have diabetes.

If the bottom number reaches 100, you are at risk for a stroke, so get to a doctor or hospital emergency room as soon as possible to go on medications to bring down the number.

Having high blood pressure is like smoking, they both can cause you to age prematurely. They can take 10 years off your life.

If you have been diagnosed with high blood pressure, then it would be worth it to have your own home digital blood pressure kit to test your blood pressure several times a day. A manual kit cost as little as $16 and a digital kit cost $30 from drug stores.

Triglycerides: Your triglyceride level should be 150 or below. Triglycerides are the main form of fat in the body. Triglycerides are a type of fat the body uses to store energy. Only small amounts are found in the blood.

Having a high triglyceride level along with a high LDL cholesterol level may increase your chances of having heart disease more than having only a high LDL cholesterol level. If you eat a lot of starches (beans, rice, potato, etc.), in your diet, this number will increase.

Waist Size: A woman's waist size should be 35 inches or less and a man's waist size should be 40 inches or less. Your waist size should be half your height. If you can only remember one number, your waist size is the one to know.

Body Mass Index: It is recommended that everyone should have a Body Mass Index (BMI) of 25 or less but don't get discouraged because for African Americans this number can be higher (or 30). The BMI is used to find out if a person is underweight, normal weight, overweight, or obese.

Resting Heart Rate: Normal resting heart rates can range anywhere from 40 to 100 beats per minute. Your resting heart rate can vary with your fitness level and with age. The fitter you are, generally the lower the resting heart rate.

Your resting heart rate should be 60 for men and 67 for women if you are fit or engage in regular cardiovascular exercises.

Certain illnesses can cause your pulse to change, so it is helpful to know what your resting pulse is, when you are well. A digital blood pressure kit will also show your resting heart rate.

Recommended List of Yearly Examinations

Everyone should get a Body Mass Index (BMI) check at each health visit. If you are apparently overweight and your doctor do not say anything about it, then you seriously need to look at getting another doctor.

In this case, your doctor obviously doesn't care anything about your health or wellness and remember many or most doctors have very little information on nutrition.

Yearly Tests for Everyone
Some of the yearly exams everyone needs include:
- A complete body physical from head to toe
- A skin exam by a dermatologist (Best time to see a dermatologist is February when the skin is pale and there is no sun damage)
- A dental exam every 6 months (Get x-rays for oral cancer. Over 70% of the population has periodontal gum disease and people with gum disease may be more likely to have a heart attack, stroke, or thickening of the arteries).

Other yearly exams if you don't have a family history or underlining health issues is a Cholesterol check (bad and good); Blood Glucose (blood sugar) check; Blood pressure check; Triglycerides check, etc.

Other tests recommended include an eye exam at least every 2 years (1 year as you age) or earlier if you have diabetes or other health issues; a HIV test at least once (additional testing is important if you have risk factors); A colonoscopy (or colorectal cancer screening) at age 50 then every 10 years after that or earlier if you have family history; a hearing test at age 65, etc.

Other Yearly Tests for Women
A yearly pap smear by age 18 to 20 (21 according to many doctors), earlier if you are sexually active (after age 30, every 1 to 3 years); Mammogram by age 35-40; and women should check with doctors about bone density tests.

Other Yearly Tests for Men
Prostate exam (PSA test and digital rectal exam) by age 40 and men should have their testosterone checked for low libido at age 35 to 40. If you have health issues or family histories, get all exams sooner.

CHAPTER 11
GET SOME TYPE OF CARDIOVASCULAR EXERCISE

The more fit you are, the longer you are likely to live. Being fit usually means you engage in some type of *"cardio"* or *"cardiovascular"* exercise. Cardiovascular exercises are any type of exercise that gets your heart rate up and keep it up for at least 30 minutes or more.

Everyone should be engaged in some type of cardiovascular exercise (fast or power walking, running, aerobics, swimming, bicycling/spinning, etc.) at least 3, 4 or 5 days a week for 30 to 45 minutes (or more).

Remember if you exercise in the morning, it speeds up your metabolism more than it would if you exercise later in the day. If you suffer from allergies, be careful exercising outside first thing in the morning especially during allergy season.

Couch Potato Lifestyle

It's estimated by many experts that this will be the first generation that will not outlive their parents. The main reason is Genetically Modified foods which have no nutritional value and leading a sedentary (sitting posture) lifestyle.

A sedentary lifestyle or *"the couch potato lifestyle"* has contributed to over 200,000 PREVENTABLE deaths a year. The leading causes of death for people with heart disease, cancer, stroke, kidney disease, liver disease, and diabetes are most strongly influenced by lifestyle.

Some easy ways to add physical activity to your daily routine include:
- Park the car farther away from your destination.
- Get on or off the bus several blocks away.
- Take the stairs instead of the elevator or escalator.
- Take fitness breaks instead of cigarette or coffee breaks. Walk, stretch or do some office exercises.
- Perform gardening, yard work, heavy house cleaning, or home-repair activities.
- Avoid labor-saving devices (turn off the self-propel option on your lawn mower or vacuum cleaner, and hide all of your TV remotes).
- Exercise while watching TV. For example, use hand weights, a stationary bike or treadmill, stretch, or perform body-weight exercises such as crunches, push-ups and squats.
- Keep a pair of comfortable walking or running shoes in your car and office. You'll be ready for activity wherever you go.
- Walk while doing errands.

What to Do Before Starting an Exercise Program

Before starting any type of regular exercise program see your doctor first to make sure your body can take working out.

Remember to always start off slow then work yourself up over the next few weeks and months to a more intense form of working out, if and only if, you are in shape for that type of workout.

If you have been sedentary for some time, try exercising in water. Water aerobics are excellent for those who are overweight or who find walking or running difficult.

Know The Dangers of Working Out in a Gym
Fitness gyms have memberships for $20 or $30 a month and you don't have to sign a contract. LA Fitness bought out Bally's. Also check out YMCAs or other neighborhood gyms. But be careful when working out in a gym.

Some of the dangers of working out in a gym include _underqualified staff_ or physical trainers (untrained staff members pretending to know what they are doing); _Bacterias on equipment_ (including exercise mats so bring your own or clean off mats) and in showers (always wear shoes); and _faulty equipment_ (people has been paralyzed from using faulty equipment at gyms so pay attention and don't exercise when you are sleepy or too tired).

Warm It Up
Make sure you warm up before exercising. Your warm-up is just as important as your workout, however, with busy schedules, people forget to stretch and heat up their bodies. Many just settle for a few toe-touches which can leave them in pain or injured.

A good warm-up will provide increased flexibility and will activate the necessary muscles for training and competition. It also speeds up your blood flow and causes your core temperature to rise, which will prepare you to train at your highest level. Good preparation makes for a great workout.

Sweating Too Much
You may not believe it, but the excessive sweating by athletes is one of the leading health problems that they experience.

During sports, athletes automatically experience sweating that sometimes makes them lose too much water from their body causing them not only to feel exhausted and drained, but other health problems as well in the long run.

Dehydration is one of the symptoms you can experience if you sweat too much. If you sweat for over an hour, or if you are an athlete that engages in an extensive workout, you will need a natural wide range of minerals and vitamins.

You can take an electrolyte stamina mineral supplement from a health food store or drink a type of sports drink (Gatorade, Powerade, etc.) with electrolytes. However, be careful of these drinks because they contain sugars, even the low-calorie drinks have a high amount of sugars.

You will also need a double or triple amount of antioxidants as compared to normal individuals to guard yourself of potential free radicals that are produced during exercise or training.

Preventing Soreness
Getting sore after exercising will not only keep you from continuing to exercise, it might make you stop all together. Therefore, to prevent soreness remember to use natural remedies for soreness versus the over-the-counter creams that will eventually leak into your blood system and cause your body to become toxic.

For instance, always keep Epsom salt by your bathtub to use when you go home from the gym and for muscle cramps rub pure, unprocessed olive or flaxseed oil into your muscles before and after strenuous exercise.

Ask the Right Questions
It's time to re-evaluate your routine. Are your goals realistic? Are you trying to attain an unhealthy weight?

Do you need more focus on cardio or strength training? These are questions you need to ask yourself, and you can get help with the answers from experienced trainers.

Once you re-examine the flaws of your fitness training program, you'll understand why you're not achieving the personal fitness goals you created. Research acceptable weight loss or gain, find cookbooks meant for your diet, and set your schedule for workout times that are manageable.

Have You Reached a Plateau?
A plateau happens when you are no longer experiencing a positive change. But it's probably not your fault, since the majority of people reaches plateaus and don't know what to do.

Most people arrive at a plateau because of lack of knowledge. They use the limited amount of information they have to power through workouts that are so similar day in and day out.

Pushing through your plateau might be as simple as changing the order of your exercises. If you repeat the same exercises each day, not only are you going to bore yourself to death, you are going to bore the heck out of your muscles as well.

Try doing the same moves in a different order, so your body doesn't know what to expect next.

The Right Way to Lose Weight

Being overweight is caused most often by overeating and under-exercising. Excessive weight can increase the risk of heart disease, high blood pressure, some forms of cancer, diabetes, and gallstones.

In order to lose weight, you must exercise. When you look at the people that are successful at losing weight and keeping it off, they are active, plain and simple.

Losing weight too quickly can suppress the immune system. Vital electrolytes, especially potassium, can be dangerously depleted, placing you at high risk for heart arrhythmia or heart attack.

Why You Need to Keep A Food Journal
Do you even know what you are eating? Eating high fiber foods, low-fat foods, and exercising on a regular basis is a healthful way to lose weight. If you want to lose weight, it might be vital to keep track of everything you put in your mouth via a food journal.

The idea is to be accountable for everything you eat to deter you from mindless snacking and overeating. Focus on nutrient-rich foods. Changing food habits and keeping excess weight off will be easier to maintain if a weight reduction program is undertaken on a gradual basis.

You should only lose a half, one or two pounds a week, which means women should eat 1600 calories a day and men 2,000 calories a day.

If you reach a plateau, women can take it down to 1,000 - 1,200 calories a day and men to 1,600 calories a day. Never go below 1,000 calories a day because then you are starving yourself.

If you go down to 500 calories a day, you will probably kill yourself.

How To Flatten Your Stomach
A woman's waistline should be 35 inches or smaller and a man's 40 inches or smaller. To get a flat stomach a good colon cleanser can help jump-start weight loss, an obvious way of shrinking your middle.

Fat that is stored around the middle is known as *"beer belly"* or *"love handles."* It doubles the risk for a host of diseases including stroke, heart disease, and cancer.

Why fat around your waist is bad for you:
- The fat around your waist tend to be more active in producing hormones and chemical messengers that cause inflammation throughout the body.
- Belly fat, deep inside the abdominal cavity, is near the liver, and the hormones and chemicals produced by abdominal fat go right to the liver. Increased fat in the liver, called *"fatty liver syndrome,"* is a risk factor for insulin resistance, which in turn is linked to type 2 diabetes and triples the risk for cardiovascular disease, hypertension (high blood pressure), and abnormal cholesterol levels.
- Also having fat around your waist squeezes your organs causing them not to work properly. Remember your organs work as a team. If one organ gives out, they all give out and you will die.

Why Yoga is So Important to Your Health
Yoga is one of the most essential exercises to engage in. Yoga can prevent middle-age spread in people of healthy weight and promote weight loss in those who are overweight.

Experts have recognized that consistent yoga regardless of whether it was practiced vigorously or not was the only physical activity consistently associated with attentive eating.

If you're eating mindfully, chances are you're eating more slowly. And if you're eating slowly and paying attention to what you're doing, you're going to be more apt to notice when you're feeling full.

For many beginners, the practice of yoga can seem confusing, even intimidating. Maybe you think you're not flexible or fit enough to try it. Well, don't be discouraged. The great thing about yoga is anyone can do it, young and old, athletes and couch potatoes.

In addition to increasing flexibility, studies show that yoga can alleviate problems linked to many illnesses especially cancer.

While engaging in yoga, the most important thing is to protect the joints, especially knees, hips, lower backs and wrists. You need to avoid doing anything that causes pain or discomfort. Then work to modify what needs to be modified.

Most gyms offer yoga classes or you can go to YogaFinder.com to find teachers in most nations of the world. To find yoga poses with specific therapeutic benefits, go to YogaJournal.com.

CHAPTER 12
GET PLENTY OF REST

The body uses sleep as a means of healing itself. So if you are sleeping poorly or if you have insomnia, you might have a hard time rejuvenating or renewing your life.

Insomnia may be caused by anxiety, stress, depression, too much caffeine, overeating, food allergies, numerous health conditions, and the use of stimulating drugs.

The first step in overcoming insomnia is to establish healthy sleep habits.

Keep a Regular Sleep Schedule

1. **_Go to Bed the Same Time Every Night:_** To get plenty of rest, the goal is to establish a *"nightly ritual."* You can establish a nightly ritual by going to bed the same time every night. Choose a time when you normally feel tired, so that you don't toss and turn. Try not to break this routine on weekends, when it may be tempting to stay up late. If you want to change your bedtime, help your body adjust by making the change in small daily increments, such as 15 minutes earlier or later each day.

2. **_Wake Up at the Same Time Every Day:_** If you're getting enough sleep, you should wake up naturally without an alarm clock. If you need an alarm clock to wake up on time, you may need to set an earlier bedtime. As with your bedtime, try to maintain your regular wake-time even on weekends.

3. **_Nap to Make Up for Lost Sleep:_** If you need to make up for a few lost hours, try to take a daytime nap rather than sleeping late. This way you will not disturb your natural sleep-wake rhythm. While taking a nap can be a great way to recharge, especially for older adults, it can make insomnia worse. If insomnia is a problem for you, consider eliminating napping. If you must nap, do it in the early afternoon, and limit it to thirty minutes.

4. **_Fight After-Dinner Drowsiness:_** If you find yourself getting sleepy way before your bedtime, get off the couch and do something mildly stimulating to avoid falling asleep such as washing the dishes; calling a friend; or getting clothes ready for the next day. If you give in to the drowsiness, you may wake up later in the night and have trouble getting back to sleep.

Make Your Bedroom Sleep Friendly

1. **_Keep Noise Down:_** If you can't avoid or eliminate noise from barking dogs, loud neighbors, city traffic, or other people in your household, try masking it with a fan or recordings of soothing sounds.

2. **_Keep Your Room Dark and Cool:_** Even dim lights, especially those from TV or computer screens, can confuse the body clock. Heavy curtains or shades can help block light from windows, or you can try an eye mask to cover your eyes.

3. **_Make Sure Your Bed is Comfortable:_** Is your bed big enough? You should have enough room to stretch and turn comfortably. Make sure you have a good mattress. When deciding on a mattress, take 10 minutes to lie on the mattress in the store before buying. If you sleep on

your side, you need a softer mattress. If you sleep on your back, you need a more firm mattress.

4. **Turn Off the Television:** Many people use the television to fall asleep or relax at the end of the day. However, you might need to get the television and even stereo out of your bedroom because it stimulates the mind, rather than relaxing it.

5. **Reserve the Bed for Sleeping:** Don't associate your bed with any type of work. Use your bed only for sleep. That way when you go to bed, your body gets the clue, it's time for sleep.

Know When to See a Sleep Doctor
The goal is to recognize when you need to see a sleep doctor such as when you have persistent daytime sleepiness or fatigue; Loud snoring accompanied by pauses in breathing; Difficulty falling asleep or staying asleep; Unrefreshing sleep; Frequent morning headaches; Crawling sensations in your legs or arms at night; Inability to move while falling asleep or waking up; Physically acting out dreams during sleep; and falling asleep at inappropriate times.

Other steps you can take to make sure you get plenty of sleep is try to stay away from big meals at night. Try to stop eating 2 to 3 hours before sleep.

If you don't get enough sleep, you can add on unwanted pounds because you will crave the bad or unhealthy carbohydrates the next day and for several days to come.

You also want to avoid alcohol before bed; Cut down on your caffeine (sodas, coffee, teas, etc.); and quit smoking because nicotine is a stimulant.

If you are still sleeping poorly after taking the steps in this chapter, there are nutrients that can help. The idea is to support your body's ability to fall asleep quickly and then stay asleep until morning.

Melatonin, a hormone that regulates the body's sleep-wake cycle, can promote drowsiness. It has been used successfully to improve sleep quality in older people with insomnia and help night shift workers adapt to different sleep schedules.

The goal is to detoxify your body, mind, and spirit while learning new eating habits while you exercise and get enough rest and sunlight.

Once you do this, you can make every moment count, not only for yourself, but for the people you live with, work with, and care for.

Once you know the basics of healthy living, you can start taking charge of your health and your life. Remember *"You Can't Be Wealthy if You are Not Healthy"* and *"Your Health is Your Wealth!"* So read this book as many times as it takes to rejuvenate or renew your life.

I hope you enjoyed this book as much as I enjoyed writing it. This is the **third** and final book of a 3-part empowerment book series. The first book dealt with family and community empowerment and the second book will teach you how to start or grow your own business.

All three books will teach you *"How To Take Control of Your Own Life,"* so I recommend that you buy all three books for your entire family.

ABOUT THE AUTHOR

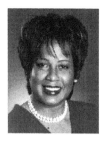

"We Can Sit Back and Watch as the World Goes By or We Can Find Opportunities to Make it Better!"
  -Cathy Harris

Cathy Harris is an Empowerment and Motivational Speaker, Health and Wellness Expert and Genetically Modified Organism (GMO) Food Expert. She launched the National Non-GMO Health Movement and is a wealth of knowledge when it comes to moving forward.

She is known as a woman in the business of uplifting and empowering her community and is an expert on many different topics including family and community empowerment, health, youth and adult entrepreneurship, writing/publishing, workplace discrimination, whistleblowing, domestic and international traveling, law enforcement, politics, media, aging, beauty – just to name a few.

She is known for her guerilla marketing style by means of forums, radio interviews, e-broadcasts, web postings and newsletters. As the author of several paperback and e-books, her non-fiction line of empowerment books has received rave reviews by everyone who has read them.

Cathy is a veteran and lives in Atlanta. She is available for lectures, seminars and workshops at http://www.CathyHarrisSpeaks.com. For more empowerment information join the mailing list and buy other books by Cathy Harris at http://www.AngelsPress.com.

CATHY HARRIS
LECTURES, SEMINARS & WORKSHOPS

http://www.CathyHarrisSpeaks.com

If you have enjoyed this book and want more assistance on how to move forward, consider attending one of Cathy's lectures, seminars, or workshops.

Lectures, seminars, and workshops are planned for the U.S. and internationally. You can benefit from a half, full, or several days of Cathy's lectures, seminars, or workshops. She will gladly travel to your city and meet with your group.

Be sure to sign up on her website at:

Angels Press
Cathy Harris, CEO
Speaker, Author, Trainer
P.O. Box 5288
Atlanta, GA 31107
Phone: (770) 873-2072
Website: http://www.angelspress.com
Email: info@angelspress.com

OTHER BOOKS BY CATHY HARRIS

The Cathy Harris Story
The Failure of Homeland In-Security
Flying While Black
Police Interactions 101
Domestic and International Traveler's Survival Guide
Recession Survival Guide
Workplace Survival Guide
Discrimination 101 (Volume I & Volume II)
How To Write A Book
My Hair, My Crown, My Glory
Politics 101
Cancer Cures
A Woman's Guide to Buying a New or Used Vehicle
(Part I & II)
A Self-Help Guide to Empowering Your Family and
the Entire Community (Series 1)
A Self-Help Guide to Starting Your Own Business (Series 2)

ARTICLES BY CATHY HARRIS

Diabetes 101
How To Engage in a Complete Detoxification Program
How To Gain Back Your Mental Clarity by Eliminating
Heavy Metals
How To Publish a Digital Book (E-book)
How To Gain Funds to Finance Your Business
How To Survive Unemployment
How To Set Up a Legal Defense Fund for False Imprisonment or
Wrongful Workplace Termination

3-PART EMPOWERMENT BOOK SERIES
Series 1, 2, 3

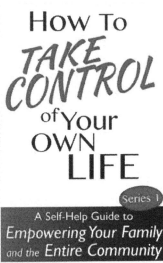

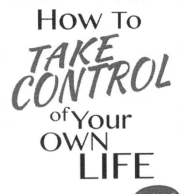

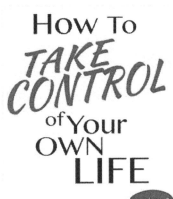

Made in the USA
Charleston, SC
24 July 2013